COMPREHENSIVE CONDITIONING FOR KARATE:

On-Mat, Strength and Conditioning and Mental Programming

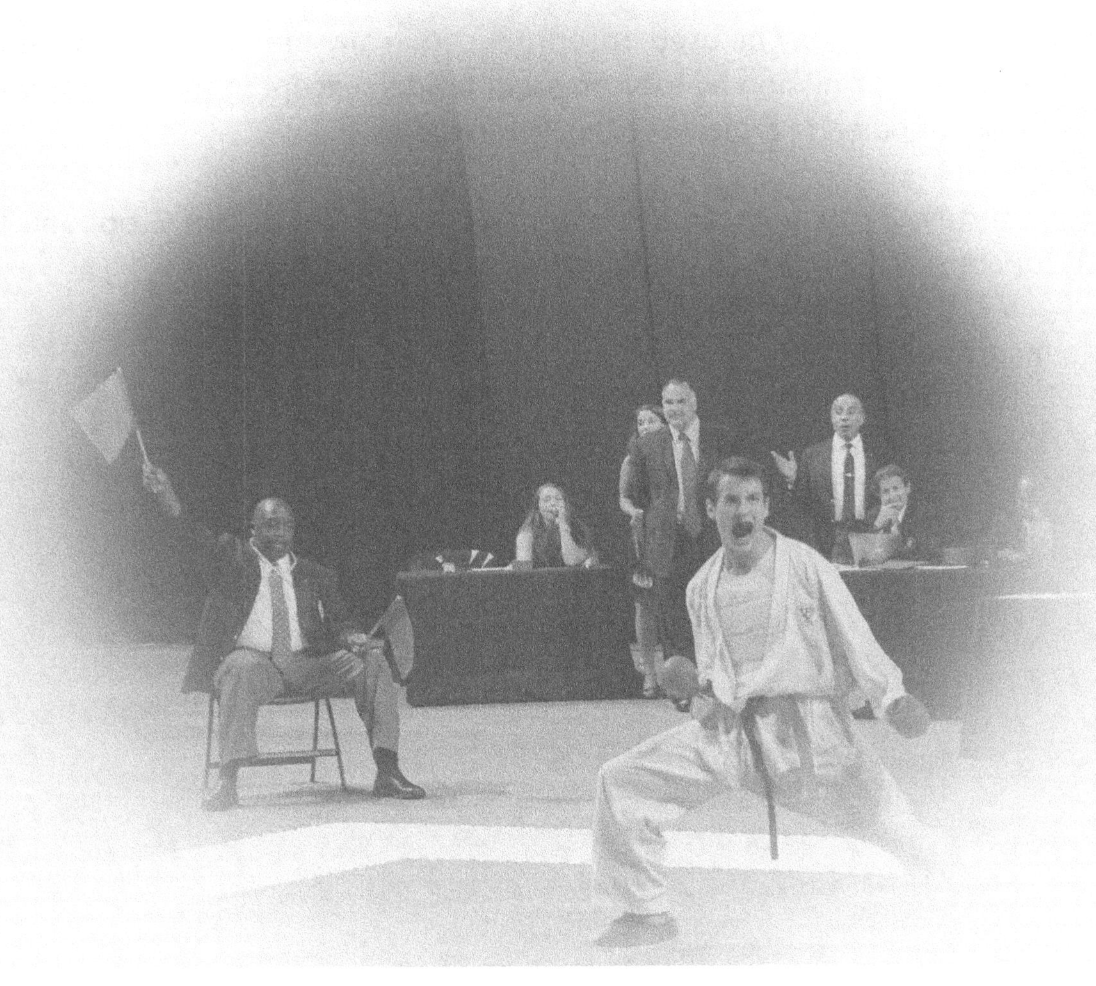

Library of Congress Cataloging - in - Publications Data.
 McClellan, Tim, and Jepperson, Doug
Comprehensive Conditioning for Karate: On-mat, Strength and Conditioning, and Mental Programming

Photos courtesy of the authors. Special thanks to Jihone Du, Jon Groot and Tom Scott, for consenting rights to name, image and likeness use.

Budo Incorporated
2815 E. Libra Street
Gilbert, AZ 85234

DEDICATION
TO SENSEIS AND TEAMMATES

SENSEIS:
A Sensei can change the mechanics of a punch or kick, and help you win a tournament. **A great Sensei can change your life.**

THANK YOU to our great Sensei's, who changed our lives:

TIM MCCLELLAN THANKS:
Doug Jepperson, Christophe Leininger, Dan Sisson, Riki Adamcik, Ray Hughes, Marlon Moore, Chuck Coburn, Hiroshi Allen, Tom Palen, Tawni McBee, and Rick Savagian.

DOUG JEPPERSON THANKS:
Rick Hobusch, Joe Sheeron, George Kotaka, Akira Fukuda, John DiPasquale,. Tom Scott, Walt Evans, John Groot, PhD, Butch Balingit, Ray Hughes

TEAMMATES:
A good teammate/training partner is more valuable than gold

TIM MCCLELLAN THANKS
Jeff "Freight Train" Dodge, Jihone Du, Simeon Ekrissin, Fred Erickson, Jason Berbaum, Kyle Harder, Mark Meyer, Madieyna Diouf, Doug Corlew, Hiroshi Allen

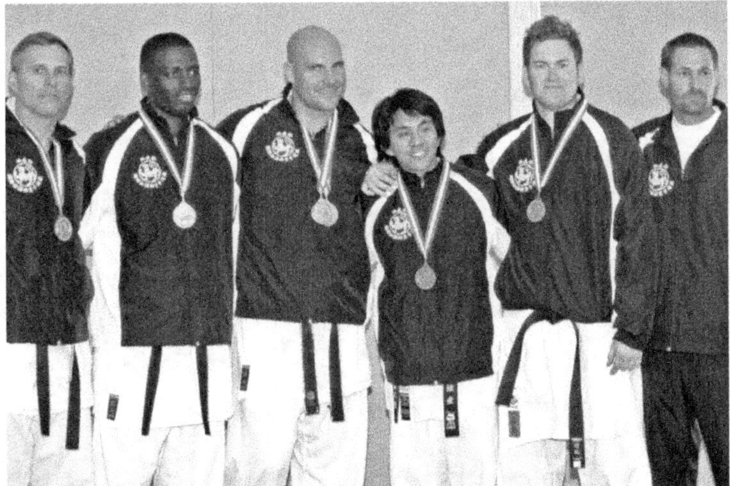

DOUG JEPPERSON THANKS:
Joe Sheeron, Rick Hobusch, Pat Burden, Bob Burden, Tito Fordman. Randy Oyama, Ray Smith

CONTENTS

1

Introduction

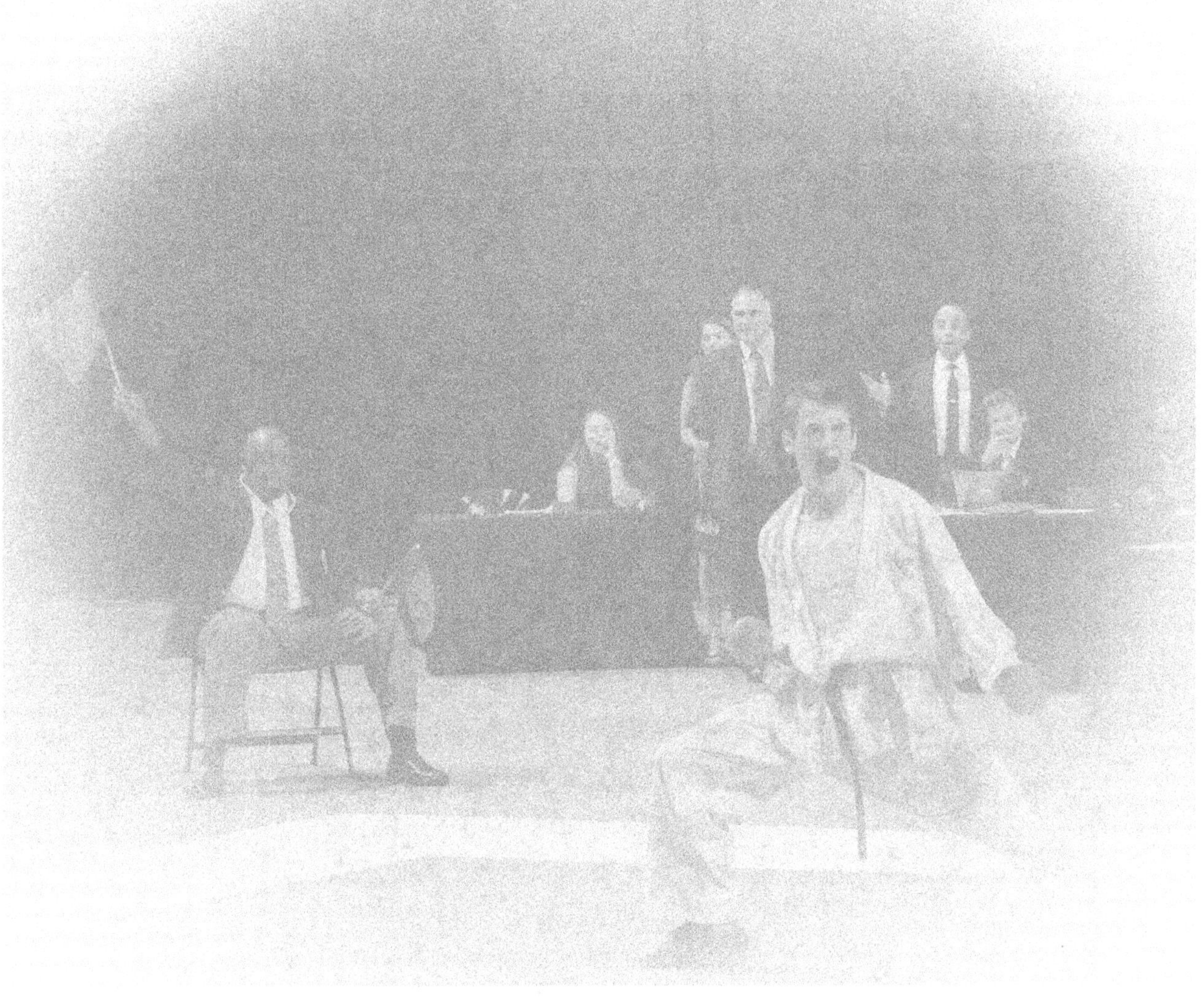

The roots of karate lineate back thousands of years. Over that span of time, it has been many things to many people. Initially it was a means of unarmed self-defense against the samurai warriors, who were privileged to be able to carry a sword while others were not allowed to, according to law. For others it was a means of learning "the way," meaning an enriched philosophical means of life. Many have used the art as a vigorous method of promoting better health, stamina, and vitality. Others have utilized it as a way to teach toughness and self-discipline. Today it has evolved into a very popular sport, as evidenced as its inclusion in the Tokyo Olympics in 2021.

Throughout this entire time, tradition and respect have been mandated essential components of "the way," of karate students and practitioners. As such, the old masters are the most revered, and their methods are typically followed by students without change or question. While this has led to honoring and respecting the masters at a high level, it has left many of today's Olympic and world-class competitive karateka at a level of training that has not evolved as it has in other sports. To put it into perspective, imagine NBA superstars LeBron James or Steph Curry doing no strength and conditioning or effective regenerative methodologies to prolong their careers and increase their productivity, because they are following the training protocols used by James Naismith when he designed the game of basketball in 1891. It would never happen. Today all professional and Olympic athletes and even most high schools are affording their athletes the benefit of having a full-time Strength and Conditioning professional to aid in their pursuit of excellence.

Unfortunately for many, karate has lagged far behind the progressive ways of sports science. Somehow the ideal of honoring the forefathers of karate became an anthem to ignore science and remain in the dark ages comparatively to the training of other athletes. It may be illustrative to tell a story, rather than complain about the "old ways."

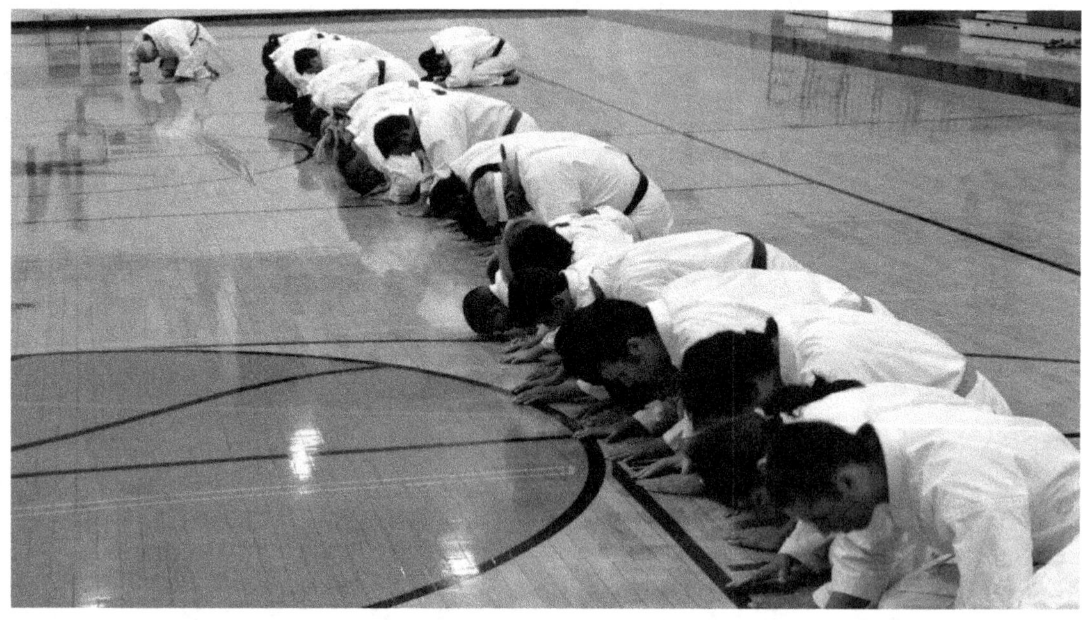

I was visiting a town recently and we wanted to find a good pizza place, so our group looked at reviews.

I found one that sounded like traditional Italian pizza. So, we decided to try it out, and upon examining a menu I noticed a claim that this pizza joint had not changed its recipes in over 50 years.

I took note because this reminded me of some of my buddies out there trying to keep the karate the same as it was 50 years ago. I decided to investigate this pizzeria and see if there were more similarities, and guess what? They claim they use "Old World Traditions."

I wondered if this was a good thing.

They use an old brick pizza oven that grandpa brought from the old country brick by brick. They used the same tomatoes as grandpa. But I know that there are modern pizza ovens with precise temperature control. Whereas the old brick oven has hot and cold spots that can sometimes burn one edge of the pizza or leave one edge not cooked as well done. And grandpa's tomatoes, well that farm in Italy has long since been made into a condo complex. And some big food conglomerate purchased the name of that original tomatoes, and now they use tomatoes grown in Florida.

Today we run faster, jump higher, live longer more active lives, build more efficient engines and yes, we know more about baking than our ancestors did. The debate is only made possible because taste and memory are subjective. It may not sound romantic and at the risk of stealing away the mysticism of pizza or karate, now is the Golden Age of Pizza, and now is the Golden Age of Karate.

Do not worry, native Italians will not be offended because today's pizza is better than yesterday's pizza. They might be more progressive than many of us. Look at what they are doing in karate. Have you seen Luigi Busa, two-time World Champion, and Olympic Champion in sparring? Or how about multiple time World Champion Luca Valdesi in kata? These are Italians and they are not cooking yesteryear's pizza. Instead, they are using the latest in technology and human development to train their karate athletes.

Let us go back to our pizza shop one more time and the idea of fifty years of an unchanged recipe. Even if that were possible, is it desirable to do something for half of a century and not learn anything new?

Further, while this pizza joint has changed nothing in 50 years, the pizza customer has changed.

Could this in any way compare to marching up down the floor, military style, doing the same old-school step and punch, over and over again, as was done hundreds of years ago, a punch, by the way, you would never use in real life or competition.

Is it me or do you see a comparison to "traditional karate?"

We should all maintain respect for the original art, respect the predecessors, while also respecting science, education, and adaption to progressive methods. This refers not only to the physiological, but also to the psychological training methods. An athlete is simply incomplete without both.

When Sir Francis Bacon published in his work, *Meditationes Sacrae* (1597), the saying: "knowledge itself is power", he expressed his idea that gaining and conveying knowledge is the key to influence, and therefore power.

The purpose of this book is to therefore try to help Sensei's, coaches and athletes to understand how to create an effective and fully comprehensive strength and conditioning and mental training program, specific to today's evolving karate athlete.

Strength Training **2**

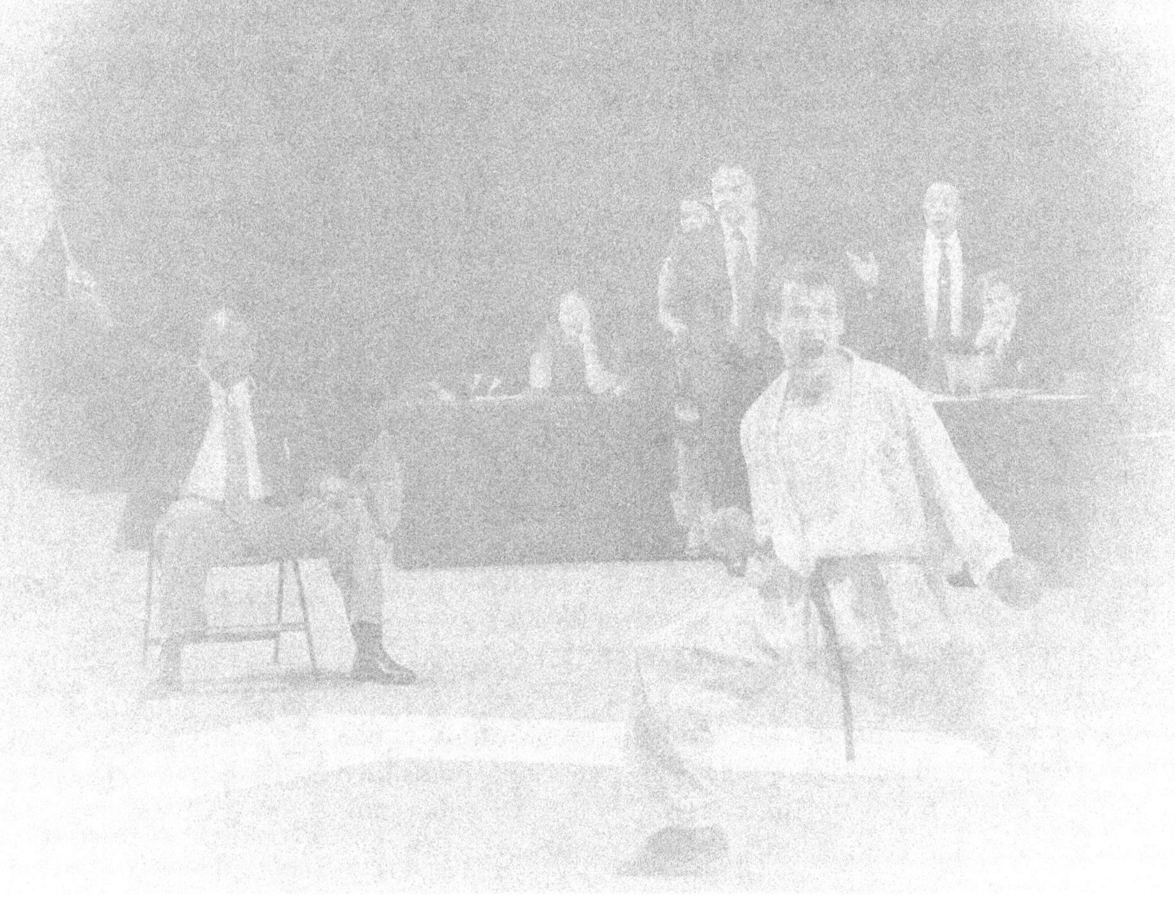

THE RATIONALE FOR STRENGTH AND CONDITIONING OFF-MAT

A growing (and somewhat concerning) trend in the field of performance enhancement is social media stars selling their "magic programs." You know the ones: "do these five weight training exercises and Rafael Aghayev will personally come to your home, give you all of his World Championship medals and post that you are his karate master". Those are obviously bogus claims and not the focus of this section, because the fact is undeniable that by far, the largest percentage of performance gains will be made on the tatami mats, not on the bench press. We have no way to estimate what percentage of performance gains are made on-mat versus off-mat, but it's got to be an exceptionally high number, like 85 percent or higher for gains being made as a result of training sport-specific techniques. There is no substitute for out working others on the tatami.

That being said, EVERY KARATE ATHLETE SHOULD BE TRAINING PROPERLY IN THE WEIGHTROOM, AND IN OFF-MAT CONDITIONING MODALITIES. Matches at any level are won by a small percentage of difference between competitors. Think of Luigi Busa's 1-0 win in the Olympic Games. Karate athletes are so close in ability typically that one point is the difference between the winner and loser of many matches. If the work in the weightroom and on the track can furnish just a little bit more speed, endurance, or energy to score that one point, it is time well spent. Our goal isn't to list just another "magic program", but rather to educate readers so well that they can create a match-changing protocol, based off their individual needs.

Here are the reasons why karate athletes can significantly improve their performance in an off-mat strength training program.

1. **PROPER TRAINING INCREASES POWER.** Power is force applied over a period of time. Think of it as initiating a blitz or retreating from one. The more explosive the first few steps are when attacking, the greater likelihood for success. Karate athletes want as much power as they can acquire. This can be garnered by increasing the force they can produce, decreasing the time it takes to produce that force, or better yet, a combination of both. Proper strength training can alter both traits, the amount of force produced and how quickly that force is maximized. No other means of training can do that.

2. **PROPER TRAINING ENHANCES TOP END SPEED.** Think of pure speed as the time when a sprinter leaves the drive phase and hits top speed. Limb speed is critical in karate, for punches, kicks, attacks, and retreats. In this sense it is not much different than sprinting. All world class sprinters lift weights because it is well known that speed up to 60-meter bursts can be improved through proper strength training.

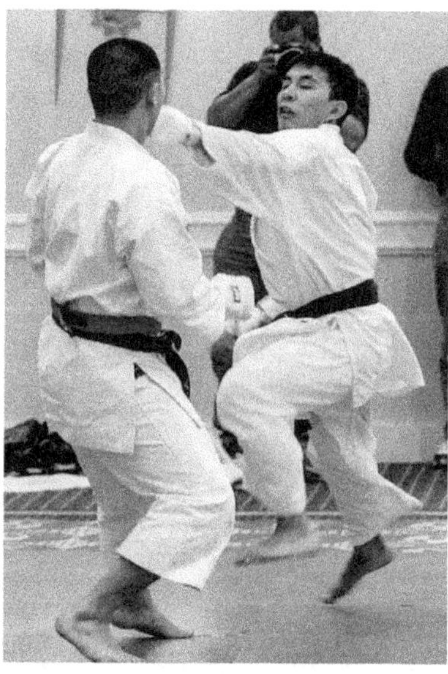

3. **PROPER TRAINING INCREASES MOVEMENT ECONOMY.** The more powerful one is, the less effort is required to initiate a desired movement pattern. Additionally, fewer motor units are called upon to activate muscle. Movement becomes much easier, and less fatiguing. The stored energy is available later in matches and tournaments, when opponents with less

movement efficiency are experiencing a decrease in performance, caused by fatigue.

4. **PROPER TRAINING DECREASES OVERUSE INJURIES.** View overuse injuries not merely as having done too much. View them as having a neurological and muscular system that can't keep up with the desired workload. Increasing strength will prevent higher levels of fatigue and the working muscles can handle the stress without that stress impacting tendons and ligaments like the patellar tendon, causing patellar tendonitis, which is too common in karate athletes.

5. **PROPER TRAINING INCREASES ENDURANCE.** Let's say you're a 75 kg. athlete capable of doing a max squat with 75 kg, and we administer an endurance test to see how many times you can squat your bodyweight. You would get only 1 rep, not good. Now let's say we get you stronger and you can max out in the squat at 125 kg. If we re-test your endurance measure, you'd likely be able to squat your bodyweight 10 times, a tenfold increase in your endurance measure.

6. **PROPER TRAINING ENHANCES NEUROMUSCULAR ACTION.** Rate of neural recruitment of fibers, firing frequency and synchronization are all enhanced with a proper training program. Additionally, and perhaps equally important, antagonists (opposing muscle groups) shut down faster and leave the body with more energy to be explosive in the desired action. Think of strength training for neuromuscular efficiency as like candy is to our tastebuds.

7. **PROPER TRAINING INCREASES BONE STRENGTH:** Mas Oyama, and countless others have spent their lives trying to perfect an art of Koppojutsu (bone breaking). We've all broken bones in kumite. Today's competitors cannot afford the time off mat. Strength training has been shown to increase bone density, structure, and strength.

8. **PROPER TRAINING CAN IMPROVE MUSCLE BALANCE.** Almost all sports promote muscular imbalance from increased unilateral practice. It's the nature of trying to optimize performance outcome that makes us spar predominantly from our stronger side. This causes us to drive more with one leg, causing an imbalance between the legs. The same applies to retreating, punching, and kicking. In theory, every time we do gyaku-zuki with the right, we should do the same with the left, but that doesn't happen due to time and energy constraints. Dumbbell training especially promotes balance between the limbs. Further, areas such as the internal rotators of the shoulder rotator cuff are often significantly worked and strengthened through on-mat repetitions and can become overly powerful as compared to the decelerators in the cuff. These imbalances can be corrected with great success in a proper program.

9. **PROPER TRAINING CAN IMPROVE END RANGE OF MOTION STRENGTH.** The hardest part of maintaining desired mechanics in the high hook kick or roundhouse kick is not at the beginning or middle of the kick, it's at the end range, where it gets hard to hold the position of a fully abducted hip. It's an awkward range of motion for humans that we don't strengthen in daily tasks. This can certainly be improved by simply throwing more kicks, but any motion lacking strength is more effectively and efficiently strengthened with the aid of external resistance.

10. **PROPER TRAINING CAN HELP REDUCE LIKELIHOOD AND SEVERITY OF TRAUMATIC INJURIES.** This alone is reason to seriously strength train. Each year in the USA alone are somewhere between 100,000-200,000 Anterior Cruciate Ligament ("ACL") ruptures, and rates among

children and teens have trended upwards of 2% annually for decades. No serious trainee can afford nine months off training, and the rehab consists of many of the same things the athlete should have been doing to prevent the rupture in the first place. You either pay before or after.

11. **PROPER TRAINING CAN RESULT IN BODY "RECOMP".** Most athletes perform better adding muscle and losing an equal amount of fat because it gives them more horsepower and a sleeker frame. Strength-to-mass ratio can improve, and that's beneficial for health in general, as well as competitive success.

12. **PROPER TRAINING CAN INCREASE SELF-CONFIDENCE.** Seeing measurables such as speed, strength or endurance tests improve naturally causes an increased belief in one's capabilities and potential. We all feed off of success. A huge percentage of this sport is mental. Those who believe, achieve.

13. **PROPER TRAINING CAN IMPROVE MOBILITY.** This is critical for high kicks, reducing chance of injuries and aiding in movement economy.

14. **PROPER TRAINING CAN INCREASE BALANCE.** Karate athletes all find themselves in very unstable positions, like getting blitzed while attempting a high kick. Strengthened muscles can stabilize moving joints faster and more forcefully, resulting in lessened imbalance and less time out of balance.

15. **PROPER TRAINING HAS BEEN SHOWN TO IMPROVE SLEEP.** Think of sleep time as "anabolic" time, where we can repair and grow better. Compromised sleep can significantly decrease performance. Restoration and rejuvenation are critical daily to get the most out of an athlete.

16. **PROPER TRAINING CAN HELP WITH BODYWEIGHT MANAGEMENT.** Caloric burn post-exercise is often higher for those who do strength training with conditioning as compared to those who do not strength train. If done properly, this can help a competitor to have the ability to stay in a lower weight division or to cut to a lower weight class.

17. **PROPER TRAINING CAN SIGNIFICANTLY IMPROVE YOUR MATCH CONDITIONING.** Matches are usually not won at the beginning, they're decided later when competitors are more tired physically, mentally and are not capable of focusing as diligently because of tiredness. If a competitor is thinking about being tired, he/she isn't properly focused on tactics. The more conditioned one is, the higher the chances of fighting well late in the match, when many matches are decided.

18. **STRENGTH AND CONDITIONING HAS BEEN TIME TESTED.** The original karate masters lifted weights by using clay jars with sand or pebbles in the. They swung heavy oars, climbed ropes, rowed boats, did plyometric hops up steps, crawled down mats, performed thousands of pull-ups and push-ups. That was strength and conditioning. The fastest athletes in the world (sprinters) strengthen and condition. Those seeking to become instant millionaires in the NFL

(Combine trainees) pay exorbitant amounts of money to improve their physiology. Perhaps the toughest/best conditioned athletes (ice hockey players) all strengthen and condition. The best moving athletes (NBA players or NFL "skill players") all lift and condition. All of the world's highest paid athletes (professional baseball) have elaborate strength and conditioning programs. Everyone has found the same thing: better training leads to better performance.

PHILOSOPHY GOVERNING OFF-MAT STRENGTH AND CONDITIONING

Karate athletes will make much of their in-competition performance gains training in the dojo and competing in tournaments. There is no substitute for these, hence strength and conditioning workouts should be viewed as a compliment to the total training program, and not a substitute for intense work on the mat. Further, improper methods can actually be counterproductive, so training must be in alignment with karate performance goals, and not ego-driven objectives like bigger biceps or a higher bench press stat to post on social media. The goal is to optimize karate skill and/or dominate opponents. If methods are not consistent with accomplishing this goal, they should be excluded.

There are literally dozens of factors that dictate physical performance ability such as, to name a few: strength, power, speed, speed-strength, strength-endurance, acceleration, deceleration, agility, balance, body control, reaction time, anticipatory skills, etc. The list is long. That being said, performance can be boiled down in a simplistic view, to three mega-factors: technical ability, tactics, and physiology (which includes psychology since the brain is part of the body).

FIGURE 1:

Athletic Success Simplified

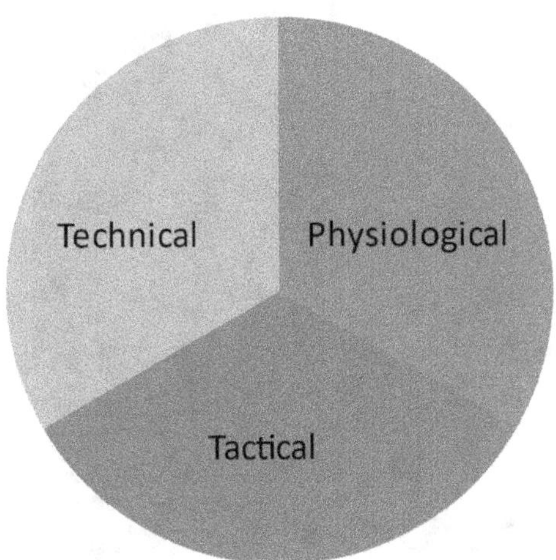

Note, without exceptions, this critical thought: you can have the most beautiful technique in the world, with great contest strategy IQ, but if you don't have outstanding physiology, you can't pull off great wins at a high level. Therefore, it is critical to have superior physiology. Without it, you cannot win.

A sound way to think about this is to consider the place a competitor has on the proverbial Bell Curve (Normal Distribution). Without getting too deep into this, a graph depicting the distribution of statistics shows where the properties lie:

1. In a classic Bell Shape

2. In symmetry

3. Unimodal (one peak)

4. 68% fall within 1 unit of the mean (average) and median (most frequent property)

5. 95% lie within 2 standards deviation units.

6. 99.7% fall within 3 units of deviation from the mean and median

Many traits fit this curve precisely, such as a person's height, birth weight, shoe size, the income distribution in most societies, the average retirement age of NFL players and even IQ and ACT test results.

FIGURE 2:

Describing the bell curve

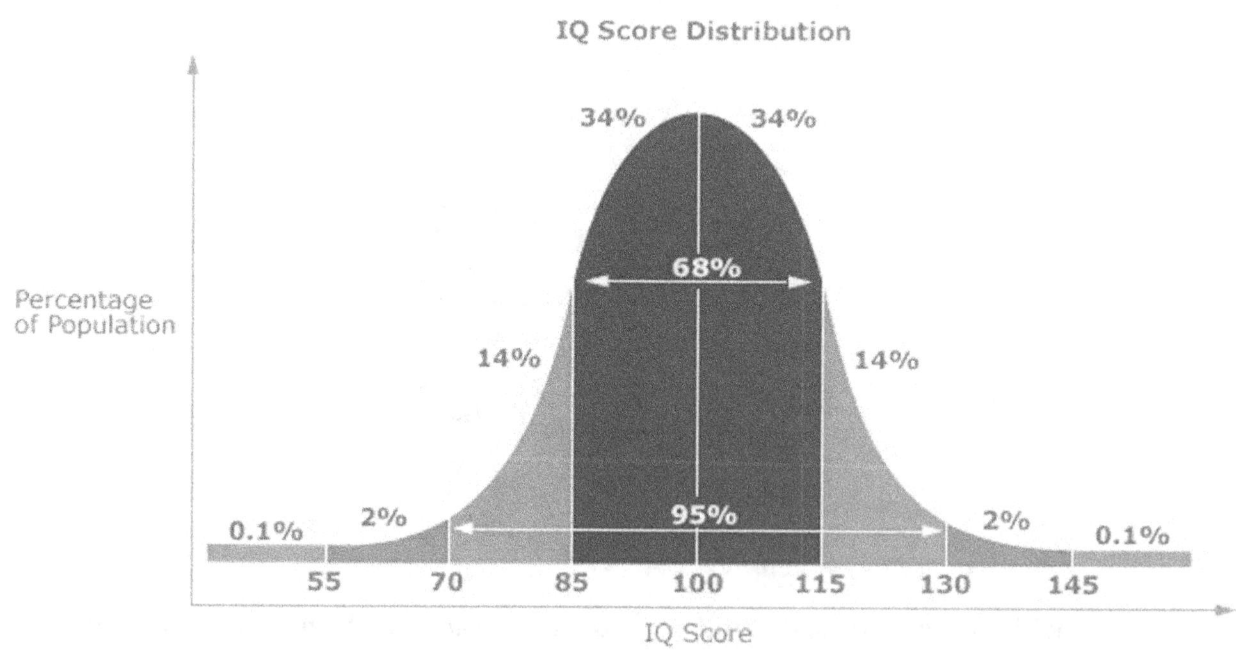

The way we can look at this through a simple analogy is this: most people (68% in the center zones) fall in the middle. You can look at this as "being normal," or as getting a "C" on

the grading scale in a class or on a test. Some people (14%) do slightly better (they are to the right of "average" by one standard deviation unit). Think of them as having achieved a "B" grade. Interestingly, 14% do slightly worse than average (they are to the left). They have earned the "D" grade. Then there are those that lie further out above average (2%) and those 2% below. Those are the outliers that earned "A" grades or "F" grades. Rarely, there are marvels, freaks, superstars, whatever you want to call them. They reside in standard deviation units farther to the right if great, or left, if awful performance-wise. This can be simply understood in the figures 3-8 below.

FIGURE 3:

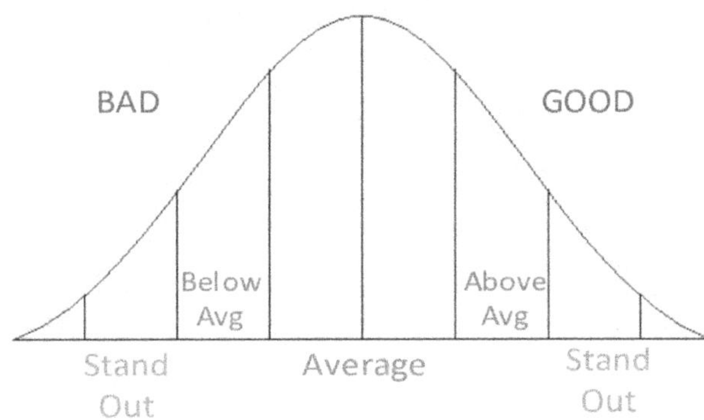

Applying this concept in coach/sensei evaluation and/or self-evaluation can be a game-changer for the karate athlete and coach. The Bell curve, as applied to karate athletes may pace an individual in one of the following Bell Curves.

FIGURE 4:

Most Karate Athletes

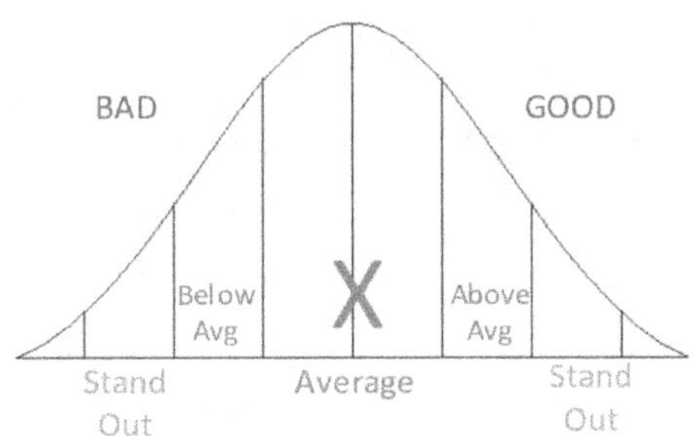

Local Tournament Champions

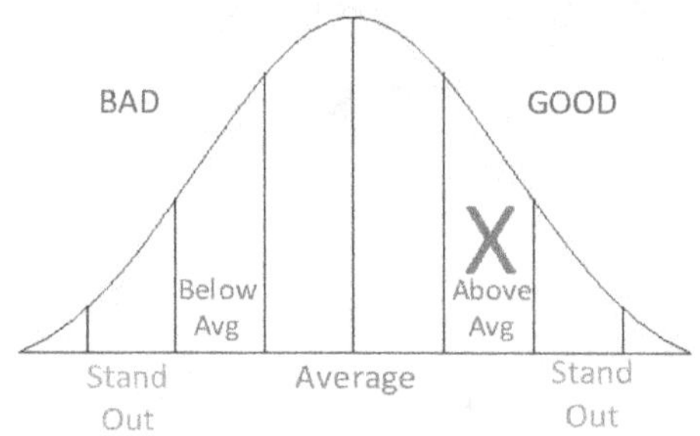

National Place Winner

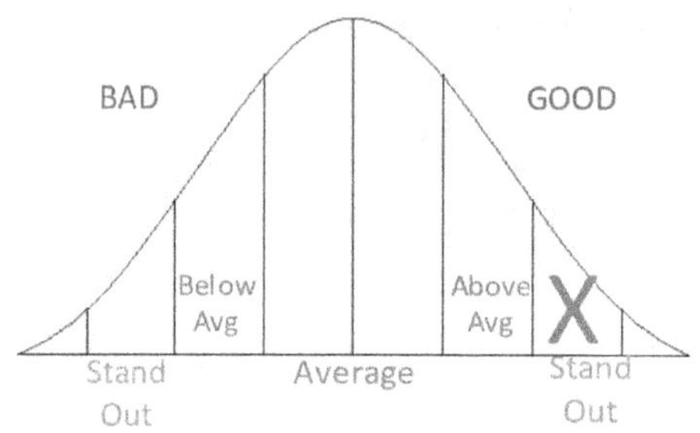

World Caliber

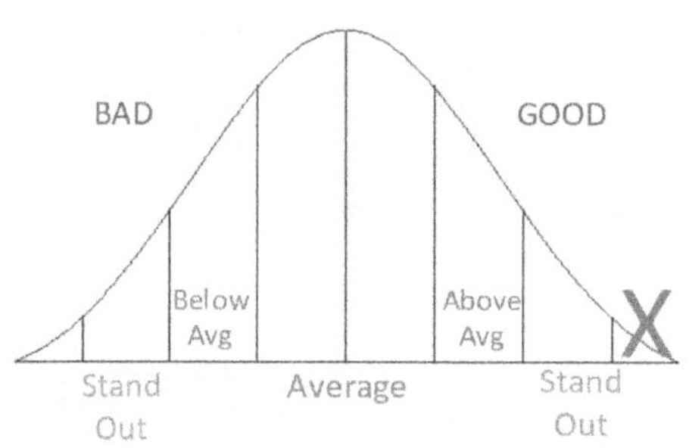

FIGURE 8:

World or Olympic Champion

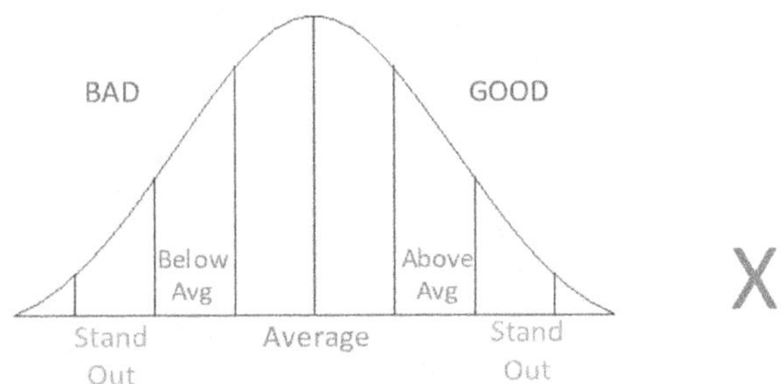

This analysis can help an individual better understand their current strengths and weaknesses. For example, Rafael Aghayev may be graded the highest score to the right on tactics, timing, IQ, experience, punching and many other things, but back one standard deviation unit for kicks (which means he is still great, but not as far of an outlier as he is in stronger areas. This assessment can help individuals and coaches determine areas of imperfection or deficiency and guide them towards planning protocols to provide a higher percentage of betterment.

With winning in mind, if you're an athlete, where do see yourself in the three mega categories: technical, tactical, physiological. If you're a coach reading this, where do you see those whom, you're coaching?

FIGURE 9:

PHYSIOLOGY

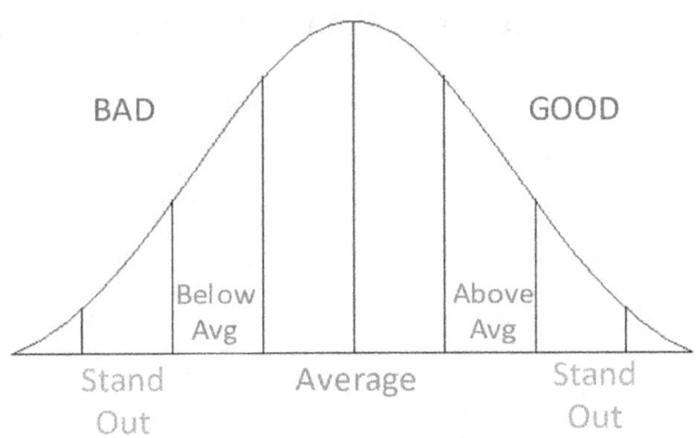

Where are you ?

More specifically, where do you stack up in the physiological traits areas that greatly impact performance in karate, such as power, speed, reaction time, acceleration, deceleration, endurance, strength, and balance?

FIGURE 10:

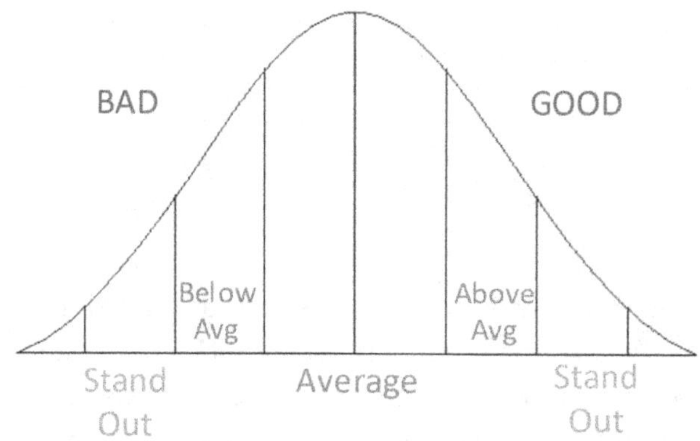

In summary, off-mat training is critical. The best athlete stands the best chance of winning. The faster athlete stands a better chance of winning. The athlete who can explode faster offensively and defensively later into a match stands a better chance of winning. The one who does all of these things typically is the champion, in most sports. Thus, karate has this in common with the NFL, NBA, NHL, MLB etc.

You now know where the elites are, and hopefully have accurately projected where you are. If you need to move over a little to the right on this Bell Curve, keep reading.

1. **INJURY PREVENTION IS THE MOST IMPORTANT FACTOR.** Karate invites injuries. It's a brutal, contact sport. Keeping athletes healthy in non-contact sports such as running, swimming and volleyball is hard enough, let alone a sport where people punch and kick one another several hours a day, often times with revenge in mind.

   Injuries that come from excessive contact are never wanted, but somewhat justifiable as a hazard of the sport. Other injuries can come from overuse (think of these as "under strong" or "under-prepared" injuries). Injuries can also be related to improper joint function. For example, toe/foot pain and especially knee pain can be a direct result of an improperly functioning ankle. Typically we say, "my knee hurts" and throw ice on it, but that is really doing not much more than making the knee cold if the cause of the injury is ankle dysfunction. These dysfunction injuries can be lessened in number and lessened in severity, producing more training time, more matches and better ability. Proper prescription of "pre-hab" exercises can make a huge difference throughout a career.

   Overuse injuries in karate can come in a variety of forms, but most notable are rotator cuff overuse ("under strength"), knee patellar tendonitis (caused by increasing volume of training too rapidly or too much, poor foot posture, leg weakness, inappropriate mechnical stress of the knee or hip, or tight quadriceps or hamstring muscles). Attention should be given in these areas, especially if a dojo is trending to have increasing or high numbers 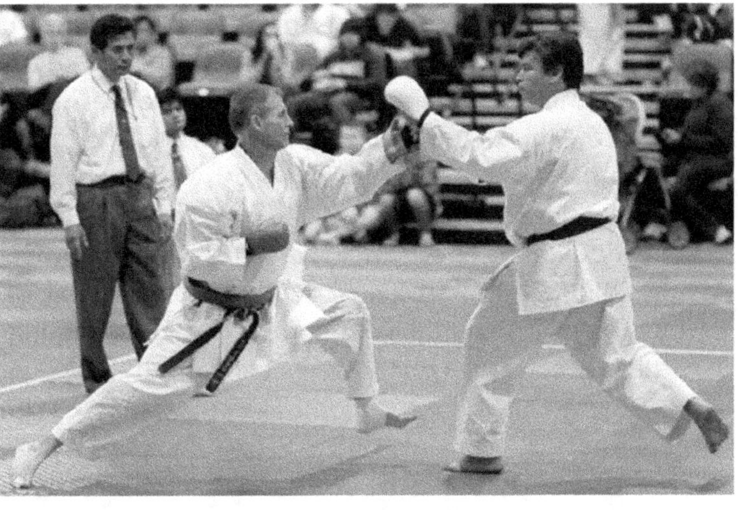 of these injuries. Thoracic spine immobility/dysfunction is another overuse injury increasing in numbers in athletics world-wide and has become an attention-grabber in the competitive sporting world, but the strengthening and mobilization of the thoracic spine inherrant in karate training has seemingly shown to reduce likelihood of injuries compared to athletes in other sports. Therefore, it is recommended to assess not only the demands of the sport and trending injuries, but also the needs of the individual before prescribing an elaborate blanket protocol that wastes valuable time with little return on the investment.

2. **TRAINING MUST BE DONE IN THE SAFEST MANNER.** Karate athletes train, simply put, to reduce potential for injuries and enhance/optimize performance. Getting hurt in the weightroom not only doesn't help the athletes from achieving those objectives, it moves them further away from them. It is therfore critical to include every safe guard possible to prevent weightroom injuries. This isn't to say that one has to live in a bubble in the weightroom and never do higher risk/ high-return exercises like cleans and squats. These are extremely beneficial choices

if they are done properly. Wheteher or not you choose to go lower risk, or slightly higher risk, great technique must be mandated on every rep, without exception, on all exercises. Otherwise, if you continue to add weight on a dysfunctional movement, all you're essentially doing is risking injury and strengthening dysfunction.

2. **TRAINING OFF-MAT SHOULD BE VERY EFFICIENT.** Athletes only get so much time and so much physical energy to train. The overwhelming majority of that time has to go to on-mat skill training. The most important factor for the strength and conditioning coach is meeting the needs of the on-mat coach. Say, for sake of example, that an athlete has a hypothetical energy expenditure level of 100. Any more expenditure pushes the athlete over the proverbial line and into overtraining, which is dangerous. Overtraining has been associated with some very serious and consequential changes in the body, including: decreased immune system function, decreased testosterone, decreased fat and carbohydrate utilization, and increased insulin resistance, cortisol, adrenal fatigue, hypothyroidism and sugar cravings. None of these are good. Combinations of these are toxic. We certainly don't want that, therefore most of the total energy (100%) should be spent on-mat, and not on the bench press, as this costs us energy, disposes us to overtraining and won't provide much benefit in performance on tournament day. As off-mat leaders we need to assess how much of that energy is taken on-mat by the coaches. In hard-driving dojos that may be 90%. In others it may be 75%. Each of these scenarios leaves us with a different amount of training energy that we can tap into off-mat. In the hard driving dojo where the Sensei/Coach is utilizing 90% of available energy, we have 10% (maximum) left for off-mat work. The off-mat work in this scenario must be reduced in volume and not too high in intensity. In the other hypothetical dojo, where the Sensei isn't burning out so much energy (75%), we can use the 25% left (at maximum), and that affords us over double the energy we have to use with the athlete in the previous example to better their physiology. The chart below depicts our ideal goal, of getting as much out of each karateka as possible, without making the mistake of overtraining. Conversely, we want to avoid doing too little, as this leaves our athletes far from their best.

FIGURE 11:

CUMULATIVE % OF ENERGY BURNED	RESULT
100+	OVERTRAINING
97-100	IDEAL TRAINING
91-96	EXCEPTIONAL TRAINING
81-90	REALLY GOOD TRAINING
71-80	GOOD TRAINING
61-70	UNDERTRAINING
51-60	
41-50	
31-40	
21-30	
11-20	
0-10	

Another way to think about this is to mirror the school grading system, as depicted in the graph below. This provides a clear, simple picture of our objectives.

Because there is an extreme time constraint, training must be super efficient. The goal is to get the maximum amount of benefit while using the least amount of effort. We need to prize quality over quantity.

FIGURE 12:

CUMULATIVE % OF ENERGY BURNED	RESULT-Grade
100+	OVERTRAINING - FAILING GRADE
97-100	IDEAL TRAINING - A+
91-96	EXCEPTIONAL TRAINING - A
81-90	REALLY GOOD TRAINING - B
71-80	GOOD TRAINING - C
61-70	UNDERTRAINING - FAILING GRADE
51-60	
41-50	
31-40	
21-30	
11-20	
0-10	

3. **PRIZE MOVEMENT SKILLS.** Simon Sinek wrote a best-selling book called *Start with Why*. Why. That's a great place to start. Why are we using our energy off-mat, if we could be using it to better our ability on mat? Next to injury prevention, the top reason why we train is to move better. Faster. More explosively. More efficient. Less taxing. Karate is all about movement. The sport has evolved from our predecessors, who were super tough, strong, frightening dudes with bad attitudes, to present day explosive, dynamic, precise super-athletes. Without great movement there can be no great success in karate.

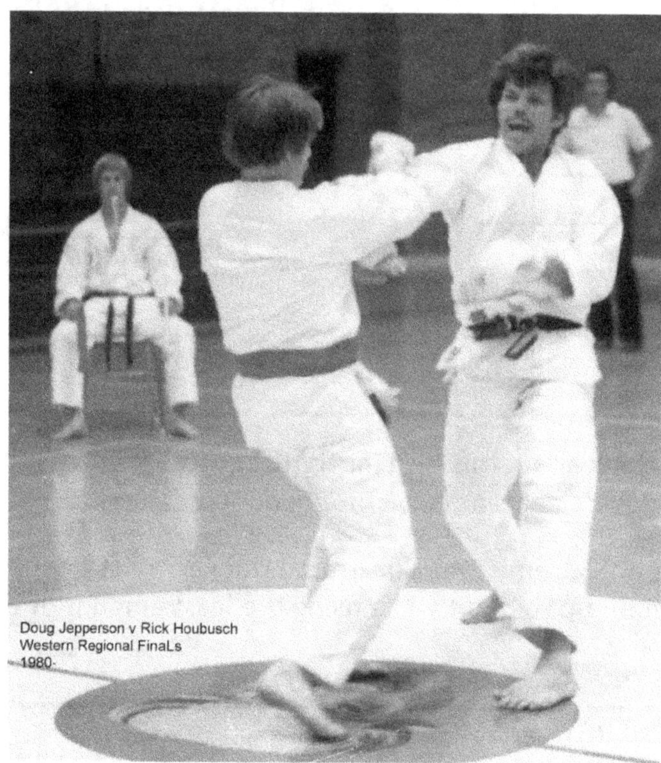

Two super tough, strong, frightening dudes with bad at-titudes.

Gray Cook is a Physical Therapist and creator of the world-renowned Functional Movement Screen (a diagnostic battery of tests to assess potential inappropriate movement restrictions due to joint/muscle dysfunction). The functional movement screen has been used extensively by the NFL, NHL, MLB, and NBA as a pro-active measure to define athletes at a higher risk of injury. Cook's philosophy is "Move well. Move often." He mandates quality movement, otherwise if you're moving improperly, you're "hitting save on a really bad document." He's right. Cook continues on with a pyramid of skills preferred for high-level athletic success. It's a little different than the ones many karateka from decades ago trained on:

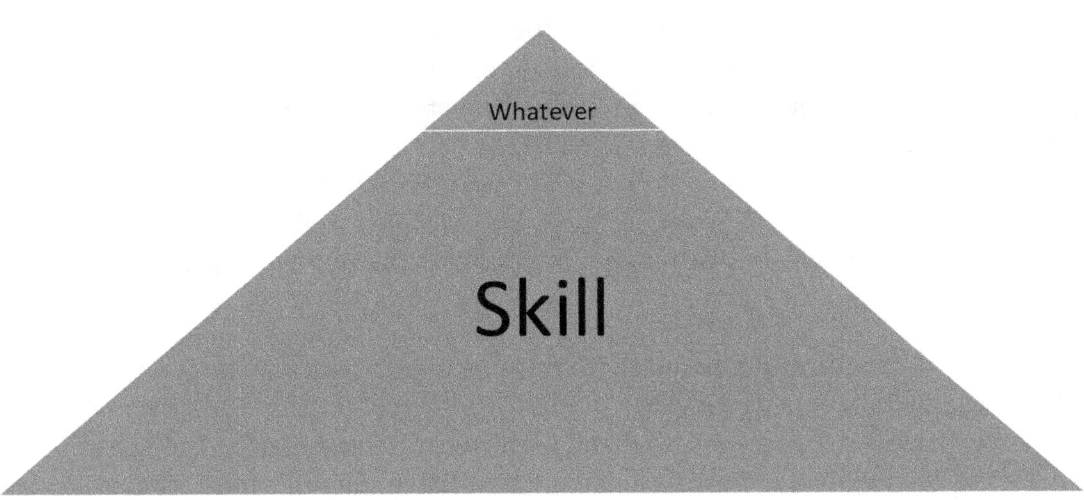

Cook's pyramid (below) for most sports more closely represents proper training objectives, where the primary goal is great movement skill, what we often call "athleticism." This is akin to the remarkable movement ability of an NBA point guard, an NFL defensive back or an all-star shortstop in MLB. Without great movement, skills cannot be pulled off at a high level.

FIGURE 14:

Among these movement objectives, first and foremost is the ability to accelerate. Acceleration gets us where we want to go. It's more than just having fast feet. History has shown us thousands of athletes with feet that looked so fast jumping rope or going through ladder footwork drills but couldn't accelerate their bodies fast enough to blitz suddenly and effectively in a karate match. This acceleration should be proficiency in moving forwards and backwards in the sagittal plane (attacking or retreating in a straight line), laterally in the frontal plane (sideways movement-for example tai sabaki, or "bobbing and weaving") and rotationally in the transverse plane: punching, dodging and countering). World-reknonwed Strength Coach Michael Boyle aptly said, " Every car goes 60 miles per hour. The difference between the Porsche and the Yugo is how fast it gets to 60 mph." We need our athletes to accelerate like Porsches, not Yugos.

Movement must be both economical, to conserve energy, and mechanically sound to optimize ability . Additionally, quality movement must also be sustainable—quality movement early in a match is useless if it becomes slow and inefficient late in a match. The top athletes are not usually the ones with the most flexibility or best three mile run time. They're the ones with the most horsepower to explode. This leads us into specificity.

4. **ADHERE TO THE PRINCIPLE OF SPECIFICITY ("S.A.I.D. Principle"):** In the most basic of explanations, training is a stimulus and a response. There is a specific adaptation to an imposed demand in training, hence, "the body becomes its function." Think of a high jumper for example. They are typically very good at being dynamic going upwards, but never outwards. In other words," you can't excel during the piano recital if you practiced on a tuba." This implies that there is a huge reward to performance via training specific to in-contest demands (mechanically, neuromuscularly, and metabolically) Conversely, there is less benefit in-contest with training that is not specific enough.

Exercises that more closely relate to sport mechanics are said to be more "functional," and should comprise the bulk of your regime. For instance, lunges, split squats, or split squat jumps more closely resemble movements inherent in kumite, than does a leg press where you are lying flat on your back in a stable position pushing hundreds of kilos of weight through a restricted range of motion.

With regards to specificity, we have to think in terms not only of replicating the motions of sport but also the velocity of contractions at times. Training methods such as using weighted vests, plyometrics, medicine balls, and elastic bands to slightly resist full speed movements can be used in a highly specific ranges of motion, and more closely resemble velocity of movement in karate. Further, using the bands to aid in increasing hand and foot speed (assisted, not resisted) is another superior training exercise to increase speed. This isn't to say that all we do off mat is mirror movements on mat. We aren't interested only in punching and kicking with dumbbells attached to our limbs. There is also a definitive and significant benefit to total body strengtheners like the Olympic lifts, squats, front squats, and Romanian deadlifts.

Again, this is simply thought of as, "the body becomes its function." A great example occurs in the track and field jumping events. The long jump, high jump, triple jump, and pole vault all require competitors to have extreme abilities in being fast, dynamic, efficient, light and to be great in acceleration…yet, rarely has anyone won the Olympic Games in two of these, and no one has ever done them all well, even though the desired physical traits are the same. This is because the body becomes the function of either jumping up, or out, or in a "hop, skip and jump," but doesn't optimize performance in all three. The body responds to how it is trained. Those that jump up often get good at jumping up. Those that jump out most often get good at jumping out. Training must be specific most of the time if possible. It must relate to karate performance for it to help karate performance.

5. **INCREASE RATE OF FORCE PRODUCTION, FORCE REDUCTION AND STATIC ABILITY:** Everyone seeks to lift heavier weights. It's fun and meaningful to do something greater than you have ever done before. But heavy and slow is not the goal for karate training. Consider the time it takes to achieve maximum rate of force. Karate is all about achieving the highest rate of force as fast as possible, as in initiating an attack, retreat, blocking or even sen-no-sen splitting. Scientists have named this "power," which is considerably different than "strength." Strength is more simply producing as much force regardless of how long it takes to do so. Powerlifters are a terrific example of this. No one cares how long it takes to move their resistance, like a maximum squat or deadlift. All that matters is how much weight they move. Power is actually defined as "explosive strength", like a shot putter, bobsled pusher or karate blitzer. The maximum force development is essential, but perhaps even more importantly is the rate of force development. Movement speeds in karate should replicate more closely those of a sprinter, and not of a powerlifter. The time difference can be immensely different in a game of acceleration and speed. Thus, the total amount of force production is a great quest, but rate of force production is even more desired. Times required to achieve maximal force in different movements are illustrated in the table below:

FIGURE 15:
from *Triphasic Training*, Cal Dietz and Ben Peterson

Time to Maximal Force Development	
Dynamic Actions	**Time (Seconds)**
Sprinting	0.08 – 0.12
Jumping	0.17 – 0.18
Shot Put	0.15 – 0.18
Powerlifting	0.8 – 4.0

A hypothetical example for our never yielding quest to increase rate of force development is shown in the following figures. In this first mythical example (figure 16), 100 units of force are developed as the peak force produced, and the time it takes to do so is in 4/100 of a second.

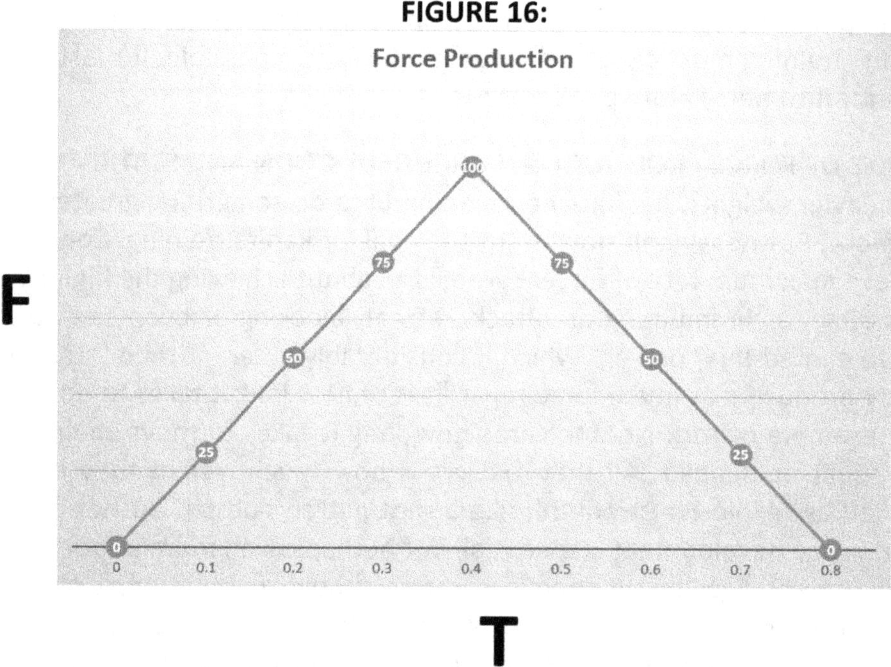

FIGURE 16:

A logical goal and huge success towards our goal of being the more powerful karateka is to produce a higher peak force in the same amount of time. In this next case below (Figure 17), 125 units of force is in 4/100 of a second. This would help us to accelerate an attack and bring more total power to our opponents. This is one way to increase power. We love to bring lots of power to our opponents. More is better.

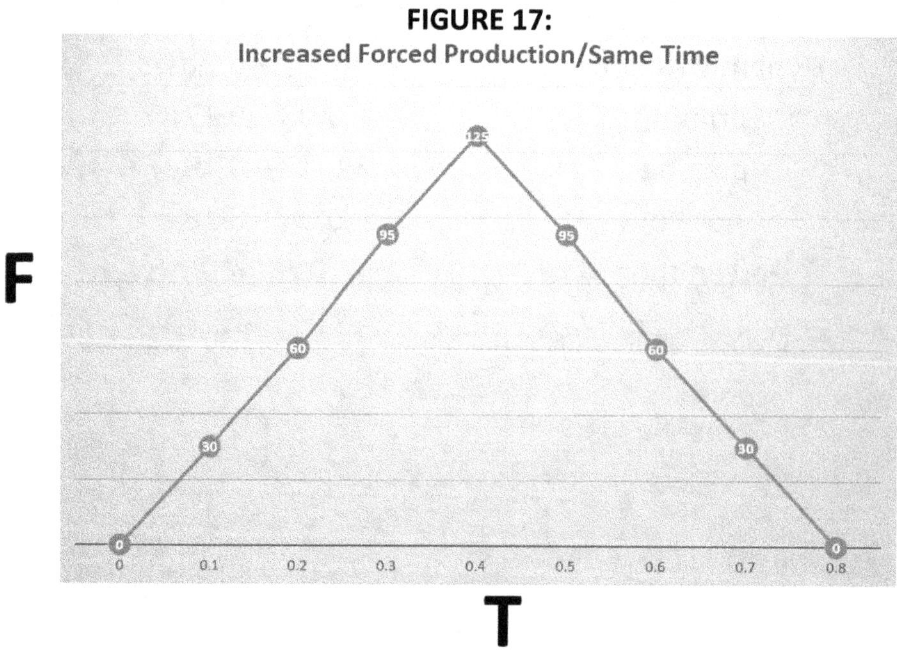

FIGURE 17:

A second way to increase force is to generate the original 100 units of force, but to do it faster. This next example (Figure 18) shows 100 units of force produced faster, in 3/100 of a second. This is like the Porsche getting to 60 miles per hour faster than the Yugo does. This is what we love to see in karateka: explosion. Speed kills.

FIGURE 18:

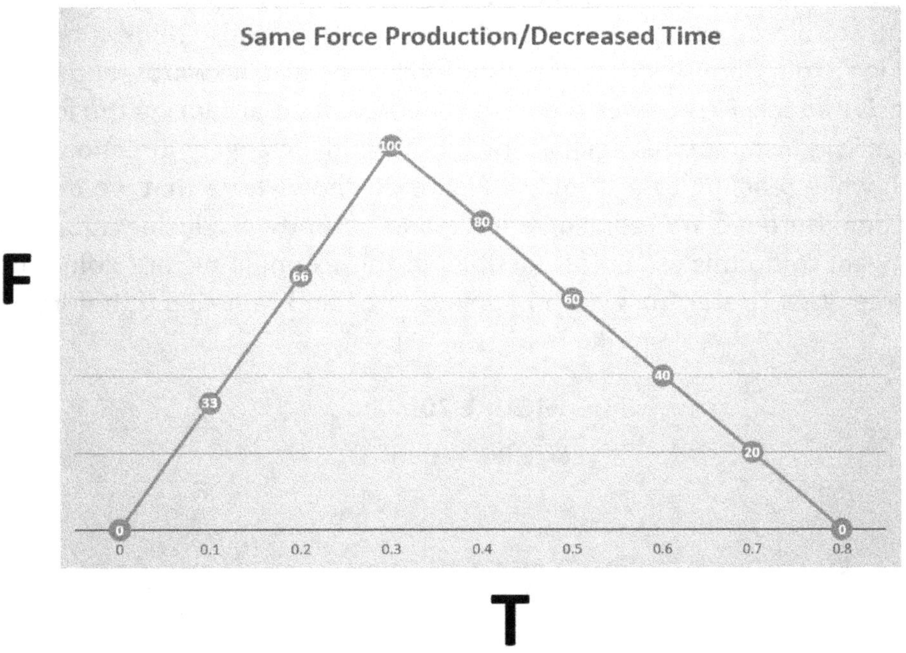

Best of all (Figure 19)— the most desired result of training, is producing greater force (125 units) at the faster rate (3/100 of a second). This is a huge force getting to our opponent faster…our goal.

FIGURE 19:

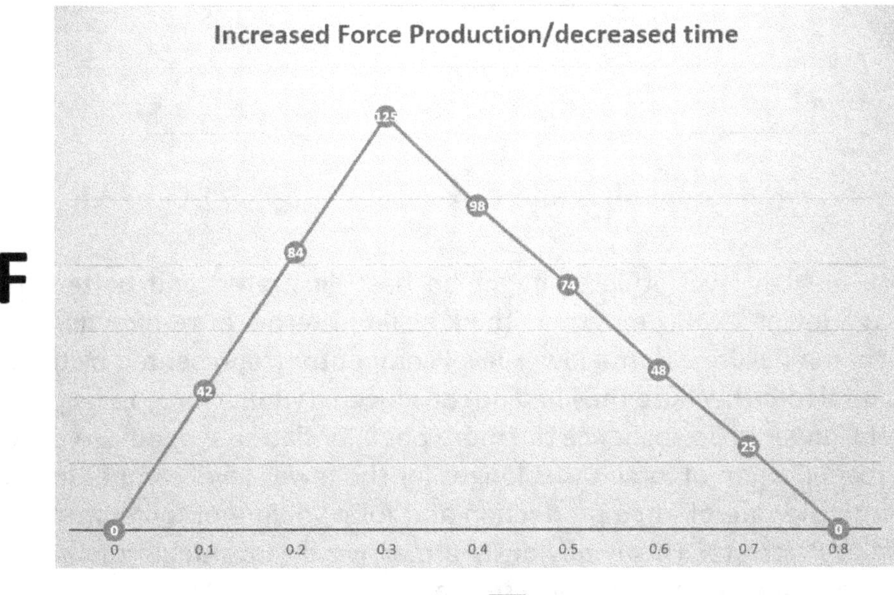

But wait, there's more to the story. Even though rate of force production is our primary trait to develop, outside of injury prevention, this isn't all that we do in kumite. We also have to reduce force, like bouncing backwards in footwork before accelerating, or changing direction. Here we must reduce the landing force before we initiate force production of bouncing forward. It is critical to decelerate as fast as possible, and with great mechanics because it precedes the next acceleration. This is called "change of direction," and is defined as being able to abruptly re-direct, without loss of body control. You can also think in terms of reducing force in blocking a roundhouse kick to the body while moving backwards, and then countering with an offensive attack. First comes reducing the force, then producing the force in initiation of the counter. This also requires agility, which is abruptly changing direction without loss of body control, while reacting to a stimulus. Figure 20 shows here that we do the inverse of force production. Here we are reducing a force and abruptly producing a force. As you can imagine, we want to do this as fast as possible. In this example we are doing the inverse of producing force. We are starting with an applied force and reducing it, before initiating our acceleration.

FIGURE 20:

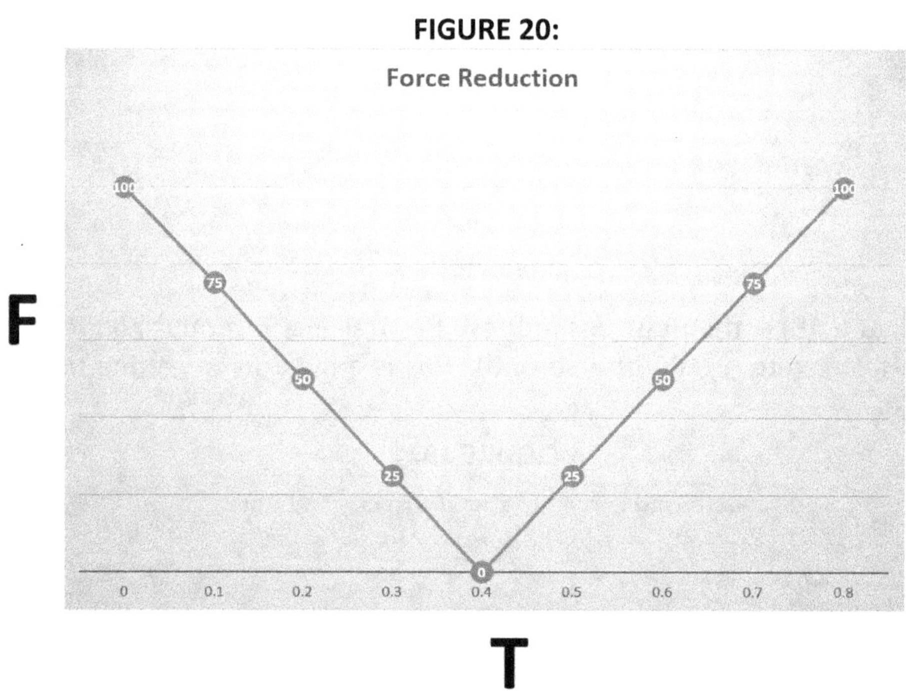

The difference in high level athletes might be best illustrated and better understood in comparison to a lower-level competitor. Think again in terms of re-directing movement. In this following graph (Figure 21), the lower-level competitor (represented by the lower line) is reducing less total force because they had not produced as much force to begin with. Sadly, it also takes them longer to do so, hence the more open, or flatter-shaped curve. Compounding matters, the reapplication of force takes longer for the lower-level competitor than the elite athlete and both the rate of force production and total volume of force produced are lower for the lower-level athlete. This is obviously a massive disadvantage for the less-explosive karateka. It is therefore critical to not only seek ability to produce force and to so fast, but also to be able to reduce force and to do that fast. Porsche. Not Yugo.

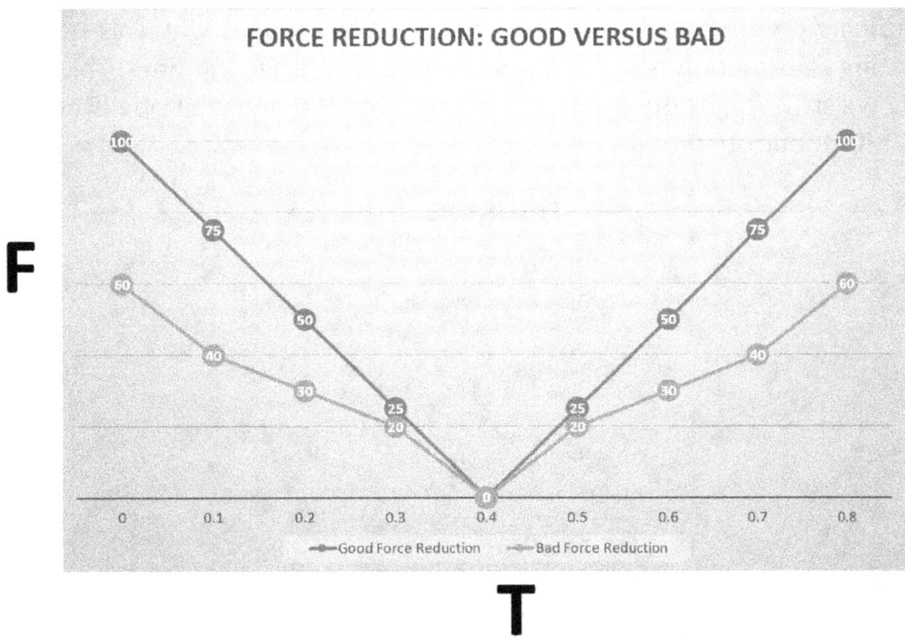

FIGURE 21:

An even slower athlete may have an even longer time in transition from the backwards bounce to the forward bounce or attack. This time difference in speed is a welcomed treat only to the more explosive competitor. Figure 22 depicts this lengthy time in re-directing.

FIGURE 22:

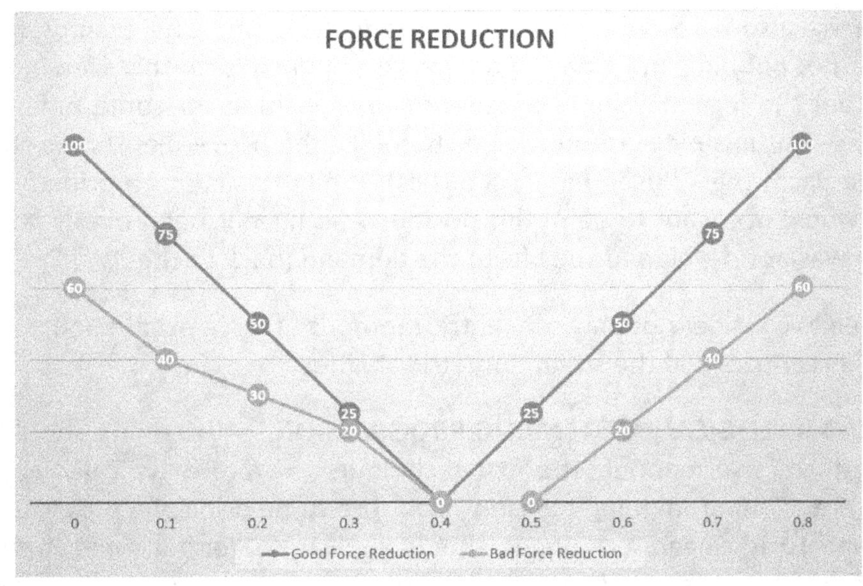

In Figure 23 we see our ideal scenario. Here the athlete is able to reduce a great force (for example, a faster deceleration) with instantaneous application of significant force and then, in an ideal training program, is able to continue to do so repeatedly. This is depicted in the athlete repeating a deceleration and abruptly accelerating a second time. This athlete has the physical body we strive to produce in our programs and the one we hope is on the other side of the bracket if it's our opponent.

FIGURE 23:

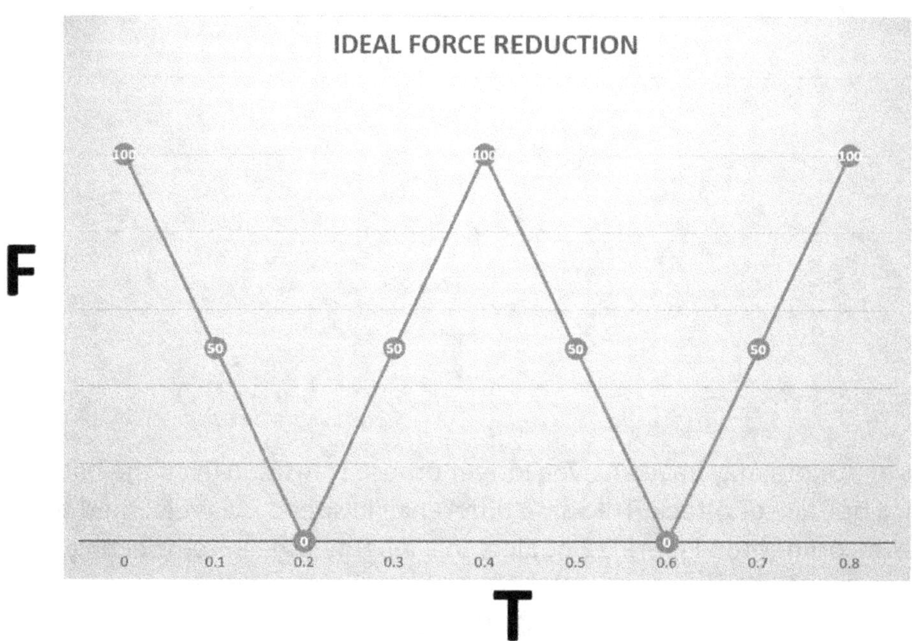

Lastly, there are also times when we can hit static positions. One example would be being stuck in a corner bobbing and weaving a barrage of punches. In this scenario the torso may be moving, but the legs may be in a deeper squat position for some time, neither flexing nor extending. This is a more isometric position (like the proverbial "horse stance" of shiko-dachi or kiba-dachi that is used in kihon basics). While this is not a primary stance used, a competitor would not want to be in this position and have it been overly fatiguing because the strength was not developed specific to the demand (back to the S.A.I.D. Principle).

Thus, we need to consider not only concentric methods of force production, but also the force reduction of eccentrics and the static isometric abilities.

6. **PROGRAM AS A "LOGICAL, SYSTEMATIC PROGRESSION."** All training should be done in a graduated, progressive manner. The first technique a karateka typically learns is a simple kizami-zuki, not a "jump spinning tornado" kick. The same principle, progressing from basics to intermediate to advanced techniques, should apply here. Yet, for some strange ("macho"?) reason, everybody always wants to test their strength right away, with little regard to safety. "How much can you bench" comes to mind here. This violates a previous principle of doing things as safely as possible.

It is therefore recommended to always use a logical, systematic progression with baseline techniques, incorporating progressions only when competency is repeatedly demonstrated. Equally important, regression techniques should be used where consistent proper biomechanics cannot be exhibited. A good example is that everyone should start a new exercise utilizing only their bodyweight, until they do so correctly and easily. At this point, they can progress logically to a very light resistance, like light dumbbells, or a weighted vest. When this is mastered, more weight can be added.

Additionally, exercise progression should go from basic movements (bodyweight squats, bodyweight split squats, step-ups, push-ups, etc.) to increasingly more difficult movements (split squat jumps, single leg Romanian deadlifts or the Olympic lifts). Once the athlete is capable of consistently demonstrating sound mechanics, weight can be slowly and steadily progressed. Progressing in weight Is important. This is called the progressive overload principle. It states that there must be a progressive stressor to the muscles to increase strength or power.

The regression protocol comes in to play when an athlete cannot master the next level they aspire to. An example here would be to cease doing improperly performed power cleans, and to resort back a level to teaching drills, like hang cleans, power shrugs from blocks and Romanian Deadlifts.

7. **UTILIZE THE PROGRESSIVE OVERLOAD PRINCIPLE.** While we strongly advocate a slower, safer progression, we must ensure that there is an increase in stress to the musculoskeletal and nervous systems. The body becomes its function, as we discussed earlier. Not only does this apply to specificity of movement, but also with regards to stress. This graph beautifully depicts what happens to our bodies when training stress is present. If the stress is too little, after rest and rejuvenation, there is little-to-no resulting benefit. Stress must increase because the same stimulus gets the same response. To get a new response (becoming faster, more dynamic, or stronger) we must have a new stimulus. Conversely, if the stress is too great, there is too much nervous system and muscular system degradation and the overtrained status leaves one worse than they had been pre-workout. But, if the stimulus is just right, we see a nice supercompensation response of betterment.

Figure 24:
from QUORA

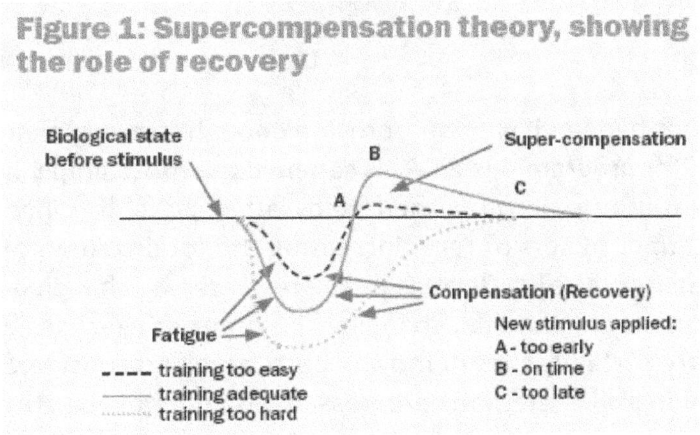

In theory, this happens day after day in this manner. In hard training there is mechanical tenson, metabolic tenson and tissue teardown. The body has been stressed and is in a "alarmed stage,' much like the model in Hans Selye's General Adaptation Syndrome. With appropriate training, rest and a flood of proper nutrients, the body responds by rebuilding itself stronger, to handle such stressors. With too much training, it cannot recover, and the body becomes inflamed and/or injured. With too little stimulus the body does not feel the need to get stronger and does not do so. It's like bath water, it has to be "just right."

Continued progression may look like this model in Figure 25:

FIGURE 25:
from athletictimemachine.com

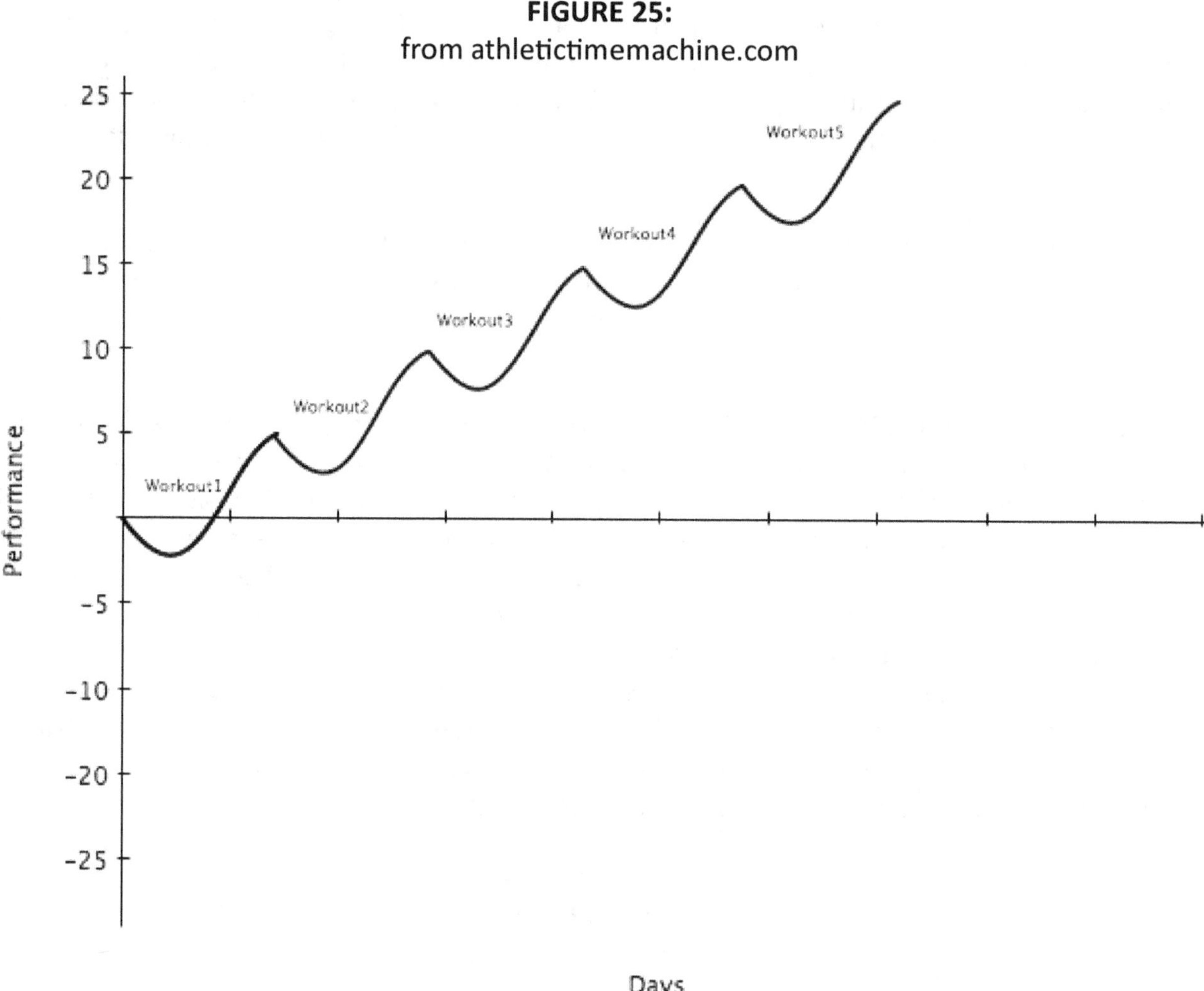

Note that this cannot happen if we don't provide enough stress. Increasing the level of stress is therefore critical for program design. This can be done most simply by adding more weight on the bar, but can also be accomplished many other ways, like increasing the number of repetitions, the number of sets of reps, increasing the total volume of the session or week, increasing the intensity of the lift, decreasing the rest interval, changing the exercise selection, increasing the frequency of the lifts, changing the order of exercises or changing the speed of the lifts. There are certainly a lot of moving parts here and considerable attention must be given to maintain a logical, systematic progression and not get too crazy while implementing the progressive overload that is essential for growth. For example, it is an almost guaranteed recipe for injury to increase both volume of work and intensity of work abruptly or too high at the same time. Leo Matveyev, referred to in the exercise physiology field as "the father of periodization," for his work in discovering optimal training methods created a hypothetical model that shows how volume of work must go down if intensity and technical focus are increased. If something isn't lowered, we get an overtrained athlete and at best there is only a decrease in performance. At worse we have a decrease in performance, an injury and a damaged psyche that can be beyond repair.

FIGURE 26:
from hmmrmedia.com

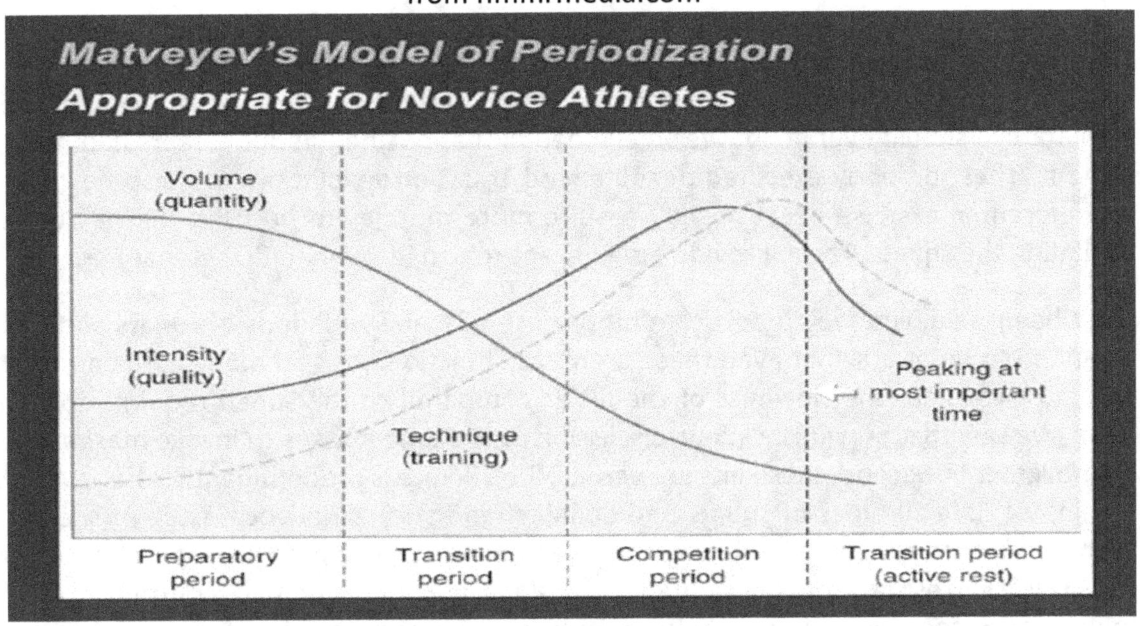

Depiction of the philosophy in designing an annual plan may therefore look like this simple model in Figure 27:

FIGURE 27:

WEIGHTROOM
VOLUME/INTENSITY CYCLING

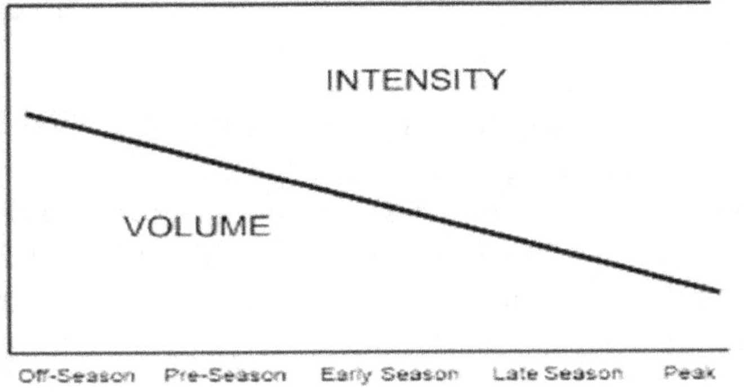

*High Intensity and High Volume do not mix

Note in this simplified version that as volume decreases, intensity can increase. We just don't want to get overzealous and start adding stress to several program design variables simultaneously.

9. **PROGRAM THE MOST PRODUCTIVE STRESSORS THAT ARE FUNCTIONAL BUT REMEMBER "SOMETHING IS BETTER THAN NOTHING."** Karate athletes shouldn't be on an off-mat program of heavy bench presses and 3-mile steady state jogs year-round. We know the S.A.I.D. Principle now and that the body becomes its function. If we ask it to run continuously and slow, and to move heavy objects while lying flat on our backs fully stabilized, we aren't most effectively preparing for the demands in kumite or kata. It is our goal to be as "functional, "as possible.

We all know by now that free weights provide more stabilization requirements than machines and are the preferred method for training. Thus, we can say squats are probably more specific, and better than leg presses, where one requires no balance and lies on their back in a position no karateka should ever be in. We've all been in that position in our careers and have never liked it. Thus, properly executed deadlifts and Trap Bar deadlifts would also be considered a preferential exercise because they require more muscles to be used than all other lifts, including the squats. These provide a significant return in a very efficient manner.

That being said, and we do advocate proper use of many variations of squats and deadlifts, we need to point out that even these aren't as "functional" as so many gurus profess. First, we must consider the slowness of the lift as compared to the speed required to punch or blitz. We saw that previously in our discussion of the time it takes to invoke maximal velocity in movements. Second, these lifts are vertical lifts. Karate is predominantly a horizontal sport. Again, we love all types of squats and deadlifts and strongly advocate use of such, but we also need more horizontal and quicker movements for development of sport-specific power. This is where resisted cords, weighted vests, sleds, and medicine balls contribute. Further, in much of karate, athletes are pushing off with more effort on one leg than the other or are on one leg at a time (this is a commonality to most sports). Thus, we need to program unilateral movements, like all types of split squats, lunges, single leg squatting movements, (even perhaps a few unilateral dumbbell bench presses to makes sure the punch we throw arrives with a little extra power). The stabilizers of the hip (the glute medius, quadratus lumborum and adductors) are called upon much more significantly in unilateral movements, than they are in heavy bilateral movements like squats, so this is yet another reason for their inclusion, or even preference in program prescription. Finally, along the lines of specificity, karateka can get into some nasty positions during matches. This is straining not only on the muscle tissues, but also on the fascia.

Two of the most renowned experts in the world with regards to flexibility as it contributes to athletic success are Ann and Chris Frederick. They wrote a fascinating book called *Stretch to Win* on the need to stretch and prepare the fascia for these scenarios where the body is immediately thrusted into very awkward positions. This is without doubt valuable in the total training program, and exercises like single leg Romanian deadlifts throughout various planes and the many variations can also be considered very appropriate and functional for karate.

Now we are all on the same page and in agreement about making "functional" choices our preference, but we must also note that "non-functional" is actually much better than nothing. It is both a wrong and illogical assumption to conclude as some "experts" do that because squats are good that leg presses are bad. Something is without doubt better than nothing. If you don't believe us, let's do an experiment using identical twins. If twin number one has to sit undertrained and sedentary, with no off-mat training, and twin number two gets to train hard on leg presses, row machines, lat pulldowns and even leg extensions, all of which are disdained by some "experts," twin number two will arrive to fight your twin with a much better body, and a competitive advantage. This athlete will also have a psychological advantage. They will perform better because they did something positive physically and mentally, and something is better than nothing. Again, we advocate specific movements, love free weights, crave function, but we must progress somehow, and non-specific movements are better than no movements.

10. **PERIODIZE YOUR PROGRAM.** Remember, gains are largely attributed to stimulus and response. A great stimulus (progressive overload) will produce a great response, an incorrect stimulus begets an undesirable response and the same ole stimulus will produce the same ole response. Programs must therefore change, ideally before the body gets too adapted to the old program and stops promoting desired growth (whether that's in gaining acceleration, deceleration, strength, endurance, or size objectives). Typically, programs are changed every 4 weeks or so. This gives the body long enough time on the current stimulus to derive sufficient benefits, but not so long that the gains gradually lessen due to familiarity. Changing programs too often does not afford the body time to adapt to the stimulus and can promote too much tissue teardown.

Perhaps the most effective means of change is to deliberately periodize the program in a system. View this as a type of ladder, where one cycle (4-week block) leads to a higher outcome, and so forth until a significantly higher level is achieved. One time-tested system that has been time-tested over decades is represented in this hypothetical model, adapted from Matveyev's original design.

The basic premise for elite athletes using this model is to do an introductory base cycle. This begins after an off-season period, following the championship season. The purpose is to bridge the gap between inactivity and harder strength training by preparing the muscles, tendons, and ligaments for increased stress. The base cycle is followed by one or more hypertrophy cycles, to gain muscle mass. The thought here is that more muscle (if done right) can help increase pure strength in subsequent cycles, because there is more muscle to move weight (including your bodyweight when moving). The strength cycles follow the hypertrophy cycle(s) with the goal of additional strength being converted to more explosive strength in the ensuing power cycles. During the power acquisition phases the magic happens, as volume is lowered, and the focus is exclusively on rate of force production and reduction. After a brief peaking phase, the competitive karateka enters in the highlight of their championship season. The athlete starts this new championship season with a transformed body, capable of dominating opponents. One step (cycle) has led to another all the way through to the championship victory.

In summary (and in simple terms) the goal coming out of a championship season is to rest after the championship season, safely reintroduce the body to increased stressors, add muscle, use the additional muscle to produce more force, make the additional force fast. Then dominate at the big events.

This is an adaptation of the Matveyev model is in Figure 28:

FIGURE 28:

McClellan's Hypothetical Model of Strength Training for Athletes

	Off-Cycle	Transitional Phase	Hypertrophy	Strength	Power	Peaking
# Cycles	1	1	1-2	2-4	2-4	1-2
Volume	0	low-moderate	very high	Semi-high/mod.	moderate	low
Intensity	0	low-moderate	moderate	high	highest	high & low
# Sets/Exercise	0	2-3	3-5	3-5	3-5 (core) 2-3 (supp)	3-4 (core) 0-3 (supp)
# Sets/Session	0	16-20	25-60	25-40	20-35	10-20
# Reps/Set	0	10-20	8-12	5-6	3-5	2-3 (core) 5-8 (supp)
Days/Week	0	2-3	4-6	3-4	2-3	2
Time/Session (minutes)	0	45-60	75-120	60-105	60-75	30-60
Rest Between Sets	0	low (circuits ?)	low	high (core lifts) mod (supp)	high	high

11. **STAY WITHIN IDEAL REP RANGES TO MEET YOUR OBJECTIVES.** All training with weights programs can alter the body. For example, many experts believe the ideal rep range per set to increase muscle mass is typically between 8-12. This is the rep range many competitive bodybuilders train in. Science shows however, that a rep range of 5-30 can also be ideal for increasing hypertrophy in some individuals. One could successfully argue that even heavy sets of 3 reps will add muscle, when compared to a program of no lifting. What's a karate athlete to do?

A simple guideline can be: 1-2 rep sets predominantly test strength and/or build neurological skill. Olympic weightlifters use these most often since the snatch and clean and jerk have a high neural component. Sets of 4-6 reps build strength, which is what many powerlifters (those who test in the squat, bench press and deadlift) choose, since that sport is more about strength and has less neural complexity comparatively to weightlifting (those who compete in the snatch, and clean and jerk). Sets of 8-12 are good rep ranges to build mass. 15+ rep sets aid endurance (most strength gains yield increased endurance anyway, as we theorized earlier.) Therefore, those needing to gain some mass (if done right, can yield gains in power) may stick to more sets of 8-12. Competitors outgrowing a weight class limit may wish to stick to a lower volume/higher intensity style workout of efficient lifts like the Olympic lifts so that they gain explosion without adding muscle and driving them up into a higher weight class.

These athletes might do 3-5 sets of 2-5 reps. The thing we need to avoid is the old-time belief of doing sets of 10 repetitions year-round to "avoid getting bigger", because this is precisely the mechanism to do so.

12. **DEVELOP BETTER BALANCE.** Karate requires extreme balance. We've all balanced precariously on one foot while throwing a high, hard kick to a tall opponent, not to mention that the opponent is trying to split the kick and run us over. In fact, we've all done that dozens of times and it has never been fun. While we can't make it fun, it doesn't have to be as threatening of a scenario if we incorporate balance training into our protocols. Items such as unilateral movement on a low balance beam (like a 2"x 4" piece of lumber can help. The objective is to not to recreate Cirque du Soleil acts, but rather to moderately increase instability and promote enhanced proprioception and balance.

13. **INCREASE CORE FUNCTION.** Everyone loves "six-pack abs," but our goal isn't to attain a desired aesthetic look of the "core". Rather, our goal is to increase balance and stability. Think not in terms of only flexion and extension exercises for cosmetic appearance, because the flexion exercises typically done are not huge contributors to the specificity of athletic performance. Think rather of trying to promote trunk stabilization and both enhanced rotation and enhanced anti-rotation. These can change performance, as they are much more specific. This should include not only the abdominals, but also the back and glutes since they attach to the spine and hips and are significant in stabilizing both.

14. **WARM-UP THOROUGHLY PRIOR TO TRAINING.** Principle 2 was all about safety. It goes without saying that we are in the weight room or on the track to enhance performance. Getting hurt from improper preparation not only doesn't aid performance, but it detracts from it. Include gentle dynamic movements throughout increasing ranges of motion. Static stretching is not forbidden. The notion that static stretching is harmful is a genuine misunderstanding of what research indicates. Besides, if it makes an athlete feel better, they should have that advantage. Foam rolling is also recommended for both physical and mental benefits.

15. **CREATE A POSITIVE CULTURE.** Decades ago, athletes had to play good to feel good. That trend has reversed itself. Athletes now need to feel good to play good. A fun weight room will provide a nice getaway from on-mat training which is hard, draining, and potentially injurious on a daily basis.

DESIGNING A PROGRAM

We now know that every karateka can benefit from a supplemental strength and conditioning program, via injury-reduction, rate of force development, enhanced posture in mechanics and many other areas. Further, we know the principles that govern exercise prescription specific to the needs an athlete has on the tatami mat. We are now tasked with putting it all together into a meaningful, productive, efficient system that hopefully turns lambs into lions.

What this looks like should change greatly from individual to individual. While we cannot detail a program for every specific need, we will show several to help create an understanding of needs assessment and resultant program prescription, so that the individual needs of all can be met. Note, we will not be explaining every exercise and/or have picture of them, as this is beyond the scope of this book, and would double its size. If clarity is needed on technique of exercises, it is recommended to purchase *Exercise Technique Manual for Resistance Training 4th Edition*, by the National Strength and Conditioning Association. This text has about four hundred pages and is written by the best in the field.

First, let's look at a sample beginner's program and recognize our aforementioned principles governing exercise prescription. This is done on a spreadsheet, commonplace in most collegiate strength and conditioning programs in the United States. Hopefully you can see the principles we previously discussed built into the program.

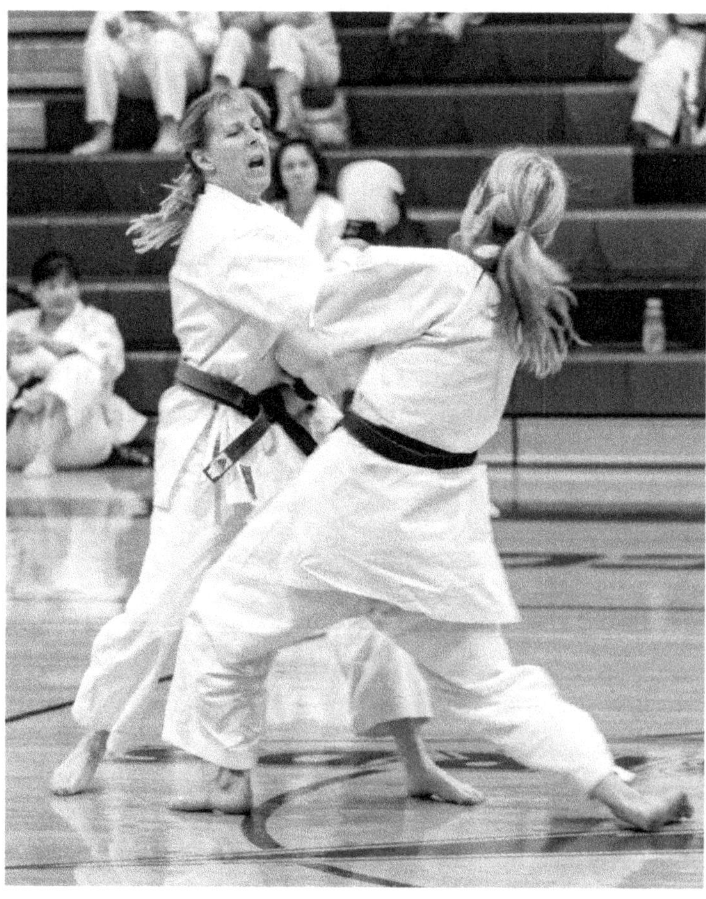

HIGH PERFORMANCE OFF-MAT TRAINING

<table>
<tr><td>PROGRAM</td><td>JILL BEGINNER</td><td>OFF-SEASON BASE CYCLE 1</td></tr>
</table>

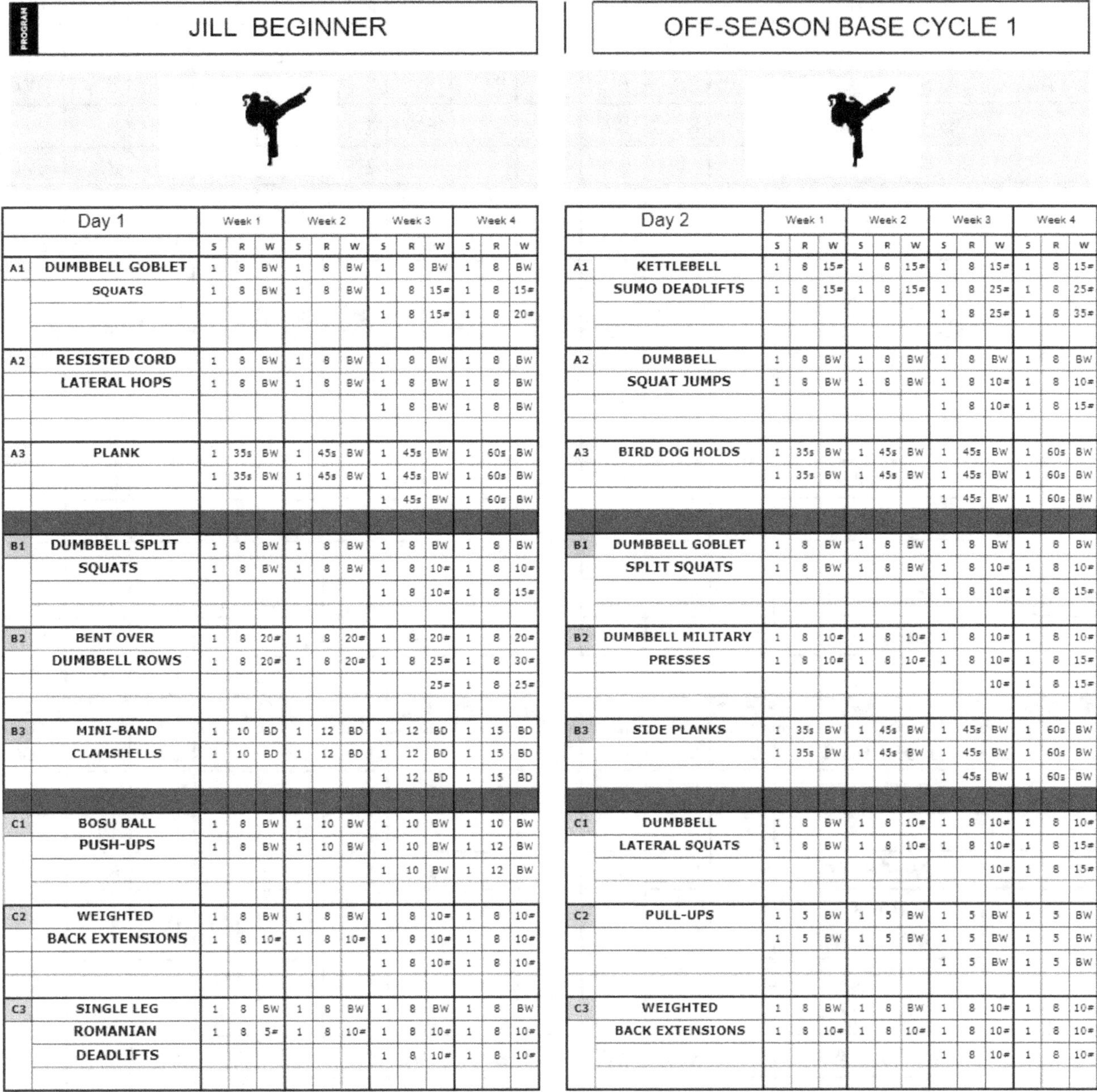

Day 1

		Week 1			Week 2			Week 3			Week 4		
		S	R	W	S	R	W	S	R	W	S	R	W
A1	DUMBBELL GOBLET SQUATS	1	8	BW	1	8	BW	1	8	BW	1	8	BW
		1	8	BW	1	8	BW	1	8	15#	1	8	15#
								1	8	15#	1	8	20#
A2	RESISTED CORD LATERAL HOPS	1	8	BW	1	8	BW	1	8	BW	1	8	BW
		1	8	BW	1	8	BW	1	8	BW	1	8	BW
								1	8	BW	1	8	BW
A3	PLANK	1	35s	BW	1	45s	BW	1	45s	BW	1	60s	BW
		1	35s	BW	1	45s	BW	1	45s	BW	1	60s	BW
								1	45s	BW	1	60s	BW
B1	DUMBBELL SPLIT SQUATS	1	8	BW	1	8	BW	1	8	BW	1	8	BW
		1	8	BW	1	8	BW	1	8	10#	1	8	10#
								1	8	10#	1	8	15#
B2	BENT OVER DUMBBELL ROWS	1	8	20#	1	8	20#	1	8	20#	1	8	20#
		1	8	20#	1	8	20#	1	8	25#	1	8	30#
										25#	1	8	25#
B3	MINI-BAND CLAMSHELLS	1	10	BD	1	12	BD	1	12	BD	1	15	BD
		1	10	BD	1	12	BD	1	12	BD	1	15	BD
								1	12	BD	1	15	BD
C1	BOSU BALL PUSH-UPS	1	8	BW	1	10	BW	1	10	BW	1	10	BW
		1	8	BW	1	10	BW	1	10	BW	1	12	BW
								1	10	BW	1	12	BW
C2	WEIGHTED BACK EXTENSIONS	1	8	BW	1	8	BW	1	8	10#	1	8	10#
		1	8	10#	1	8	10#	1	8	10#	1	8	10#
								1	8	10#	1	8	10#
C3	SINGLE LEG ROMANIAN DEADLIFTS	1	8	BW	1	8	BW	1	8	BW	1	8	BW
		1	8	5#	1	8	10#	1	8	10#	1	8	10#
								1	8	10#	1	8	10#

Day 2

		Week 1			Week 2			Week 3			Week 4		
		S	R	W	S	R	W	S	R	W	S	R	W
A1	KETTLEBELL SUMO DEADLIFTS	1	8	15#	1	8	15#	1	8	15#	1	8	15#
		1	8	15#	1	8	15#	1	8	25#	1	8	25#
								1	8	25#	1	8	35#
A2	DUMBBELL SQUAT JUMPS	1	8	BW	1	8	BW	1	8	BW	1	8	BW
		1	8	BW	1	8	BW	1	8	10#	1	8	10#
								1	8	10#	1	8	15#
A3	BIRD DOG HOLDS	1	35s	BW	1	45s	BW	1	45s	BW	1	60s	BW
		1	35s	BW	1	45s	BW	1	45s	BW	1	60s	BW
								1	45s	BW	1	60s	BW
B1	DUMBBELL GOBLET SPLIT SQUATS	1	8	BW	1	8	BW	1	8	BW	1	8	BW
		1	8	BW	1	8	BW	1	8	10#	1	8	10#
								1	8	10#	1	8	15#
B2	DUMBBELL MILITARY PRESSES	1	8	10#	1	8	10#	1	8	10#	1	8	10#
		1	8	10#	1	8	10#	1	8	10#	1	8	15#
										10#	1	8	15#
B3	SIDE PLANKS	1	35s	BW	1	45s	BW	1	45s	BW	1	60s	BW
		1	35s	BW	1	45s	BW	1	45s	BW	1	60s	BW
								1	45s	BW	1	60s	BW
C1	DUMBBELL LATERAL SQUATS	1	8	BW	1	8	10#	1	8	10#	1	8	10#
		1	8	BW	1	8	10#	1	8	10#	1	8	15#
										10#	1	8	15#
C2	PULL-UPS	1	5	BW	1	5	BW	1	5	BW	1	5	BW
		1	5	BW	1	5	BW	1	5	BW	1	5	BW
								1	5	BW	1	5	BW
C3	WEIGHTED BACK EXTENSIONS	1	8	BW	1	8	BW	1	8	10#	1	8	10#
		1	8	10#	1	8	10#	1	8	10#	1	8	10#
								1	8	10#	1	8	10#

On the left, we can see Day 1, and on the right, Day 2. Obviously, this is a two day per week program, which is great for beginners, older competitors, lower-level competitors and most everyone training for fitness. Below the day designation, we see the exercises to be done that day, and the order. Note that these are all basic, but highly productive exercises. There are no overly complex or technical lifts like snatches or clean and jerks. Safety is first. Let's zoom in...

FIGURE 30:

Day 1		Week 1			Week 2			Week 3			Week 4		
		S	R	W	S	R	W	S	R	W	S	R	W
A1	DUMBBELL GOBLET	1	8	BW	1	8	BW	1	8	BW	1	8	BW
	SQUATS	1	8	BW	1	8	BW	1	8	15#	1	8	15#
								1	8	15#	1	8	20#
A2	RESISTED CORD	1	8	BW	1	8	BW	1	8	BW	1	8	BW
	LATERAL HOPS	1	8	BW	1	8	BW	1	8	BW	1	8	BW
								1	8	BW	1	8	BW
A3	PLANK	1	35s	BW	1	45s	BW	1	45s	BW	1	60s	BW
		1	35s	BW	1	45s	BW	1	45s	BW	1	60s	BW
								1	45s	BW	1	60s	BW
B1	DUMBBELL SPLIT	1	8	BW	1	8	BW	1	8	BW	1	8	BW
	SQUATS	1	8	BW	1	8	BW	1	8	10#	1	8	10#
								1	8	10#	1	8	15#
B2	BENT OVER	1	8	20#	1	8	20#	1	8	20#	1	8	20#
	DUMBBELL ROWS	1	8	20#	1	8	20#	1	8	25#	1	8	30#
										25#	1	8	25#
B3	MINI-BAND	1	10	BD	1	12	BD	1	12	BD	1	15	BD
	CLAMSHELLS	1	10	BD	1	12	BD	1	12	BD	1	15	BD
								1	12	BD	1	15	BD
C1	BOSU BALL	1	8	BW	1	10	BW	1	10	BW	1	10	BW
	PUSH-UPS	1	8	BW	1	10	BW	1	10	BW	1	12	BW
								1	10	BW	1	12	BW
C2	WEIGHTED	1	8	BW	1	8	BW	1	8	10#	1	8	10#
	BACK EXTENSIONS	1	8	10#	1	8	10#	1	8	10#	1	8	10#
								1	8	10#	1	8	10#
C3	SINGLE LEG	1	8	BW	1	8	BW	1	8	BW	1	8	BW
	ROMANIAN	1	8	5#	1	8	10#	1	8	10#	1	8	10#
	DEADLIFTS							1	8	10#	1	8	10#

For this program, all the "A" exercises are done first, in a mini-circuit fashion. In other words, in week one, Jill Beginner would do 1 set of 8 Dumbbell Goblet Squats with only her bodyweight, followed by 8 resisted cord lateral hops, and then a 35 second plank hold. After a short rest, she would repeat the circuit one more time and she will be done with the "A" grouping. This makes for very efficient training, as compared to a weightlifter or powerlifter style session where the lifter rests 1-4 minutes between sets of the same exercise. Note that there are only 2 sets of 8 reps per exercise, so the volume is very low and manageable, and appropriate for beginners. Note also we are working the squats in the sagittal plane, and the resisted cord lateral hops in the frontal and transverse planes. We are also doing core work, through stabilization and not merely flexion, as this increases specificity. All of this is in accordance with our aforementioned principles.

When the "A" exercises are done, Jill Beginner will move onto circuit the "B" exercises. Dumbbell split squats are both highly sport-specific ("functional") and unilateral, so we are activating the glute medius, quadratus lumborum and adductors of the hips for strength and stabilization. We are combining those with bent over dumbbell rows, which include some low back isometric contraction and possibly rotation. This can help posture and balance out the overuse of forward flexion and rotation that is sometimes seen in so much daily punching. We are finishing that circuit with clam shells, which are a great resisted hip abductor movement and is specific to the strengthening of the hips in throwing high side kicks, roundhouse kicks and hook kicks. The "B" exercises are also done in two circuits, as indicated on the sheet.

Upon completion of the "B" exercises Jill moves to "C" exercises where she leads off with a very efficient upper body strengthener (Bosu ball push-ups), while stabilizing the core simultaneously. We've added great glute/hamstring/core strengthening exercises in doing weight back extensions. Lastly, she performs single leg Romanian deadlifts, a terrific hamstring strengthener that provides great balance, unilateral development, and injury prevention.

Week 2 she would perform the exact same routine, and this affords the body the opportunity to adapt, without providing too much stress. Weeks 3 and 4 however Jill Beginner progresses both the volume and the intensity (weight) in a very safe manner. Weight is added. This is our progression. This will provide productive stress and will cause an adaptation in the body we are seeking.

Moving over to day 2, we have changed the exercises so she can derive benefit from strengthening muscles in different joint angles, ranges of motion and muscular contractions. This is critical to grow as always limiting ranges to few areas leaves much room for improvement in motions not trained in. The first circuit is to teach kettlebell sumo deadlifts, and with this being an easy exercise we started out with a very mild weight right away (15 pounds). We progress to dumbbell squat jumps to increase velocity of contraction and aid in our rate of force production. The third exercise are bird dog holds, a phenomenal core stabilizer. The 2nd circuit has both upper body (dumbbell military presses) and lower body exercises (dumbbell goblet split squats), both being unilateral. The 3rd exercise in the circuit is the side plank, another great core stabilizer. Circuit "C" has us moving in the frontal plane to develop our lateral movement via dumbbell lateral squats. We also see pull-ups as an upper body strengthener and weighted back extensions that we did on day 1. As with day 1, week 2 is very much the same but weeks 3 and 4 progress in volume, load, and intensity.

FIGURE 31:

Day 2		Week 1			Week 2			Week 3			Week 4		
		S	R	W	S	R	W	S	R	W	S	R	W
A1	KETTLEBELL	1	8	15#	1	8	15#	1	8	15#	1	8	15#
	SUMO DEADLIFTS	1	8	15#	1	8	15#	1	8	25#	1	8	25#
								1	8	25#	1	8	35#
A2	DUMBBELL	1	8	BW	1	8	BW	1	8	BW	1	8	BW
	SQUAT JUMPS	1	8	BW	1	8	BW	1	8	10#	1	8	10#
								1	8	10#	1	8	15#
A3	BIRD DOG HOLDS	1	35s	BW	1	45s	BW	1	45s	BW	1	60s	BW
		1	35s	BW	1	45s	BW	1	45s	BW	1	60s	BW
								1	45s	BW	1	60s	BW
B1	DUMBBELL GOBLET	1	8	BW	1	8	BW	1	8	BW	1	8	BW
	SPLIT SQUATS	1	8	BW	1	8	BW	1	8	10#	1	8	10#
								1	8	10#	1	8	15#
B2	DUMBBELL MILITARY	1	8	10#	1	8	10#	1	8	10#	1	8	10#
	PRESSES	1	8	10#	1	8	10#	1	8	10#	1	8	15#
										10#	1	8	15#
B3	SIDE PLANKS	1	35s	BW	1	45s	BW	1	45s	BW	1	60s	BW
		1	35s	BW	1	45s	BW	1	45s	BW	1	60s	BW
								1	45s	BW	1	60s	BW
C1	DUMBBELL	1	8	BW	1	8	10#	1	8	10#	1	8	10#
	LATERAL SQUATS	1	8	BW	1	8	10#	1	8	10#	1	8	15#
	-									10#	1	8	15#
C2	PULL-UPS	1	5	BW	1	5	BW	1	5	BW	1	5	BW
		1	5	BW	1	5	BW	1	5	BW	1	5	BW
								1	5	BW	1	5	BW
C3	WEIGHTED	1	8	BW	1	8	BW	1	8	10#	1	8	10#
	BACK EXTENSIONS	1	8	10#	1	8	10#	1	8	10#	1	8	10#
								1	8	10#	1	8	10#

Let's compare and contrast the novice-type of program that Jill Beginner has, to the more complex one of Joe Advanced. Joe is a larger, more experienced kumite competitor, perhaps around 86 kilos or even larger. Joe has considerable experience in the weight room, has seen the benefits and loves this facet of the complete conditioning program. He feels his increased strength gives him an advantage over his opponents, and fact is, if he truly believes this, it probably does. Because he is elite, as a competitor, and in his approach, his program is highly detailed. Joe starts each session with a neurological activation period ("A"). Here the goal is to warm-up and prepare the body through low-level, fast feet, high coordination exercises like speed/agility ladders or jump rope patterns. There are many more ways to do this, like dot drill pads, low-level box footwork patterns and cone drills. Hundreds of drills can be invented and implemented here. There is much more to follow on this in following chapters.

Period "B" is a dynamic mobility/muscle activation sequence, such as dynamic movement sequences ("mobility drills") and can sometimes include low-stress activation exercises like glute bridges. The next period ("C") is designated not only to prepare and warm the body, but also to aid in injury prevention, most notably the rotator cuff and the ankles. After that, Joe is prepped to do serious developmental lifting, trying to positively alter his physiology. Day 1 and 3 are 3 sets of a concentrated heavy lift, complete with percentage of one rep maximum capability to ensure that he isn't choosing a weight that is too heavy or too light, while progressing. This is very important for lifters with a good amount of experience. The circuits that follow are predominantly explosion development exercises, like squat jumps, resisted cord shuffles, resisted cord lateral hops, plyometric hurdle hops, split squat jumps and medicine ball throwing. The upper body volume of work is not immense, in fact the volume is quite low, so the intensity should correspondingly be high. Note the specialization in exercise prescription, delineating rear foot elevated split squats into ones done in a knee-dominant method versus ones done in a hip dominant fashion. This is a trait of programming for very elite athletes, not a necessary concern for most karateka. Finally, note movements very specific to on-mat demands, like kick strengthening with ankle weights through both normal range of motion and deliberately reduced range of motion. These are super beneficial. They must be done slow, but if done properly, nothing can strengthen end range of motion better than them (extreme hip abduction in high kicks). Remember, this program, like Jill Beginner's, is just a hypothetical model to illustrate concepts. It's not provided as a means that all elites should train. Those having trouble making weight, older competitors and others might have more success on a lower volume program.

FIGURE 32:

Day 1		Week 1				Week 2				Week 3				Week 4				
		S	R	%	W	S	R	%	W	S	R	%	W	S	R	%	W	
A	SPEED AGILITY LADDER (if not coming from practice)	1	8		BW	1	8		BW	1	8		BW	1	8		BW	CHOOSE PATTERNS FOR FOOTWORK PREFERENCE
B	MOBILITIES:																	
	KNEE TO CHEST WALK	1	10M			1	10M			1	10M			1	10M			
	LEG CRADLE WALK	1	10M			1	10M			1	10M			1	10M			
	QUADS	1	10M			1	10M			1	10M			1	10M			
	BACKWARDS HAMSTRING	1	10M			1	10M			1	10M			1	10M			
	STRAIGHT LEG LUNGE	1	10M			1	10M			1	10M			1	10M			
	LATERAL GROIN	1	10M			1	10M			1	10M			1	10M			
	QUAD WITH AN RDL	1	10M			1	10M			1	10M			1	10M			
	HIP ABDUCTION WALK	1	10M			1	10M			1	10M			1	10M			
	HIP ADDUCTION WALK	1	10M			1	10M			1	10M			1	10M			
C	CIRCUIT:																	NO REST UNTIL FINISHED
	TUBING ANKLE DORSI FLEXION	2	10			2	10			2	10			2	10			
	TUBING ANKLE PLANTAR FLEXION	2	10			2	10			2	10			2	10			
	TUBING CLOCKWISE CIRCLES	2	10			2	10			2	10			2	10			
	TUBING COUNTER-CLOCKWISE CIRCLES	2	10			2	10			2	10			2	10			
	TUBING INTERNAL SHOULDER ROTATIONS	2	10			2	10			2	10			2	10			
	TUBING EXTERNAL SHOULDER ROTATIONS	2	10			2	10			2	10			2	10			

		1	5	50%	150	1	5	50%	150	1	5	50%	150	1	5	50%	150	
D	**FRONT SQUAT**	1	5	50%	150	1	5	50%	150	1	5	50%	150	1	5	50%	150	** BASED OFF OF 300 POUND MAX
		1	5	65%	195	1	5	65%	195	1	5	65%	195	1	5	65%	195	** BASED OFF OF 300 POUND MAX
		1	5	75%	225	1	5	79%	235	1	5	82%	245	1	5	85%	255	** BASED OFF OF 300 POUND MAX
E	**CIRCUIT:**																	
	PUSH UP ROWS	3	8			3	8			3	8			3	8			NOTE: 3 SETS OF THIS EXERCISE
	DUMBBELL SQUAT JUMPS	2	5			2	5			2	5			2	5			
	FORWARD HURDLE HOPS	2	5			2	5			2	5			2	5			
F	**CIRCUIT:**																	
	MED BALL PUNCH PASS	3	8			3	8			3	8			3	8			NOTE: 3 SETS OF THIS EXERCISE
	RESISTED CORD LATERAL SHUFFLE	2	5			2	5			2	5			2	5			FULL SPEED
	RESISTED CORD LATERAL HOP	2	5			2	5			2	5			2	5			
G	**CIRCUIT:**																	
	SINGLE LEG LATERAL DROP JUMPS	2	5			2	5			2	5			2	5			
	WEIGHTED SLOW HOOK KICK OFF BOX	2	5			2	5			2	5			2	5			ANKLE WEIGHTS NEEDED
	WEIGHTED SLOW SIDE KICK OFF THE BOX	2	5			2	5			2	5			2	5			ANKLE WEIGHTS NEEDED
	WEIGHTED SLOW FRONT KICK OFF THE BOX	2	5			2	5			2	5			2	5			ANKLE WEIGHTS NEEDED
	WEIGHTED SLOW ROUNDHOUSE KICK OFF THE BOX	2	5			2	5			2	5			2	5			ANKLE WEIGHTS NEEDED

FIGURE 33:

	Day 2	Week 1				Week 2				Week 3				Week 4				
		S	R	%	W	S	R	%	W	S	R	%	W	S	R	%	W	
A	**SPEED AGILITY LADDER** (if not coming from practice)	1	8		BW	1	8		BW	1	8		BW	1	8		BW	CHOOSE PATTERNS FOR FOOTWORK PREFERENCE
B	**CIRCUIT:**																	NO REST UNTIL FINISHED
	GLUTE BRIDGE	2	5			2	5			2	5			2	5			
	SIDE LYING HIP ABDUCTION	2	5			2	5			2	5			2	5			
	PRISONER GOOD MORNINGS	2	5			2	5			2	5			2	5			
	PRISONER SQUATS	2	5			2	5			2	5			2	5			
	OPEN GATE	2	5			2	5			2	5			2	5			
	CLOSED GATE	2	5			2	5			2	5			2	5			
	STRAIGHT LEG OPEN GATE	2	5			2	5			2	5			2	5			
	STRAIGHT LEG CLOSED GATE	2	5			2	5			2	5			2	5			
C	**CIRCUIT:**																	NO REST UNTIL FINISHED
	STANDING SCAPTION	2	10			2	10			2	10			2	10			
	SUPINE SCAPTION	2	10			2	10			2	10			2	10			
	PRONE INCLINE LATERAL RAISE	2	10			2	10			2	10			2	10			
	PLATE CIRCLES	2	10			2	10			2	10			2	10			
	TIB BAR FLEXION	2	10			2	10			2	10			2	10			
	UNSTABLE SURFACE BALANCING	2	10			2	10			2	10			2	10			

	Exercise																	Notes
D	**SUPERSET:**																	
	SIDE TO SIDE LATERAL HURDLE HOPS	2	8			2	8			2	8			2	8			
	MED BALL PUNCH PASS	2	8			2	8			2	8			2	8			
E	**SUPERSET:**																	
	FRONT FOOT ELEVATED SPLIT SQUAT	2	8			2	8			2	8			2	8			** EMPHASIZE FORWARD KNEE FLEXION OVER TOES
	PULL-UP	2	8			2	8			2	8			2	8			
F	**SUPERSET:**																	
	KNEE DOMINANT REAR FOOT ELEVATED SPLIT SQUAT	2	8			2	8			2	8			2	8			** EMPHASIZE FORWARD KNEE FLEXION OVER TOES
	DUMBBELL BENCH PRESS	2	8			2	8			2	8			2	8			
G	**SUPERSET:**																	
	HIP DOMINANT REAR FOOT ELEVATED SPLIT SQUAT	2	5			2	5			2	5			2	5			** RESTRICT FORWARD KNEE MOVEMENT AND FLEXION
	NEUTRAL GRIP CHIN-UP	2	5			2	5			2	5			2	5			
H	**CIRCUIT:**																	
	ECCENTRIC NORDIC LEG CURLS	2	3			2	3			2	3			2	3			
	WEIGHTED SLOW FRONT KICK	2	5			2	5			2	5			2	5			ANKLE WEIGHTS NEEDED
	WEIGHTED SLOW ROUND-HOUSE KICK	2	5			2	5			2	5			2	5			ANKLE WEIGHTS NEEDED
	WEIGHTED SLOW SIDE KICK	2	5			2	5			2	5			2	5			ANKLE WEIGHTS NEEDED
	WEIGHTED SLOW HOOK KICK	2	5			2	5			2	5			2	5			ANKLE WEIGHTS NEEDED

FIGURE 34:

	Day 3	Week 1				Week 2				Week 3				Week 4				
		S	R	%	W	S	R	%	W	S	R	%	W	S	R	%	W	
A	**JUMP ROPE**	5	30 S			5	30 S			5	30 S			5	30 S			CHOOSE PATTERNS TO SUIT YOUR NEEDS
B	**CIRCUIT:**																	NO REST UNTIL FINISHED
	STANDING LEG CRADLE	2	5			2	5			2	5			2	5			
	GLUTE BRIDGE	2	10			2	10			2	10			2	10			
	STANDING QUAD INTO RDL	2	5			2	5			2	5			2	5			
	LEG SWINGS	2	5			2	5			2	5			2	5			
	FORWARD STRAIGHT LEG LUNGE	2	5			2	5			2	5			2	5			
	LATERAL LEG SWING	2	5			2	5			2	5			2	5			
	HIP CIRCLES	2	8			2	8			2	8			2	8			
C	**CIRCUIT:**																	NO REST UNTIL FINISHED
	SIDE LYING EXTERNAL ROTATIONS	2	8			2	8			2	8			2	8			
	TIB BAR FLEXIONS	2	8			2	8			2	8			2	8			
	SIDE LYING INTERNAL ROTATIONS	2	8			2	8			2	8			2	8			
	SIDE LYING HIP ABDUCTION	2	8			2	8			2	8			2	8			
	QUADRIPED BIRD DOGS	2	8			2	8			2	8			2	8			
	SINGLE LEG HEEL RAISE	2	8			2	8			2	8			2	8			

	Exercise	Set	Rep	%	Weight	Set	Rep	%	Weight	Set	Rep	%	Weight	Set	Rep	%	Weight	Notes
D	**TRAP BAR DEADLIFT**	1	5	50%	200	1	5	50%	200	1	5	50%	200	1	5	50%	200	** BASED OFF OF 400 POUND MAX
		1	5	65%	260	1	5	65%	260	1	5	65%	260	1	5	65%	260	** BASED OFF OF 400 POUND MAX
		1	5	75%	300	1	5	79%	315	1	5	82%	330	1	5	85%	340	** BASED OFF OF 400 POUND MAX
E	**CIRCUIT:**																	
	RESISTED CORD LATERAL HOP	2	8			2	8			2	8			2	8			
	RESISTED CORD BLITZ	2	8			2	8			2	8			2	8			YOUR CHOICE OF COMBINATIONS
	DUMBBELL BENCH PRESS	2	8			2	8			2	8			2	8			** SEMI SUPINATED
F	**CIRCUIT:**																	
	DUMBBELL SPLIT SQUAT JUMPS	2	8			2	8			2	8			2	8			
	WEIGHTED DIPS	1	12		BW	1	12		BW	1	12		BW	1	12		BW	
		1	5			1	5			1	5			1	5			ADD WEIGHT
	SIDE PLANK	2	1 MIN			2	1 MIN			2	1 MIN			2	1 MIN			
G	**CIRCUIT:**																	
	ALT LEG LATERAL LUNGE	2	8			2	8			2	8			2	8			
	HOP TO SINGLE LEG RDL	2	5			2	5			2	5			2	5			
	MED BALL PUNCH PASS	2	10			2	10			2	10			2	10			

PUTTING IT ALL TOGETHER

So now that we know why to supplement dojo training with strength and conditioning, what principles we are wise to adhere to, and what various programs look like, how do we put it all together and create monsters?

STEP 1

First, we need to assess not only the needs of the sport, but also other factors, like the fighting style of the karateka. There will be a very detailed section later in this book in the "On-Mat Conditioning" chapter on factors to be considered when evaluating the karateka. We also need to assess the peculiar needs of the individual. Is there concern about the ability to accelerate? Is body mass too big or too small? Are backward and sideways movements where they should be in terms of both acceleration and speed? The list to assess here is long and should involve the karate coach, the athlete, and the strength and conditioning professional. The goal is to get a clear vision of what we are trying to achieve and what the end-product should look like.

STEP 2

Second, we have to determine the number of sessions per week the athlete can always make, without fail, and the amount of time needed per session. Make no doubt about this: by far, the number one factor contributing to success is the consistency and compliance in training. It is far better to plan two sessions per week for only forty-five minutes and never miss a workout, than to embark on an elaborate three or four day per week program for an hour and a half and then drop out of it because it's too much. Twice a week at 45 minutes per session for a 50-week year gives us 75 hours of betterment. Three one and a half hour sessions per week for a month and then quitting because it's too much, leaves us with only 18 hours, less than a quarter of the time the more consistent athlete completed doing shorter sessions.

STEP 3

Once we determine the amount of time per work-out and the days per week, we can start designing the protocol. There are literally thousands of exercises to choose from that can be combined into millions of different protocols. Perhaps a sound method of reasoning in teaching one how to construct programs would be to categorize movements into classifications and to draw from categories during program design. This mirrors the model of most nutritional program designs, where foods are categorized into exchange lists, such as fruits, vegetables, fats, proteins, etc. This is done to provide flexibility and increase compliance in the nutritional program, as opposed to prescribing the same foods every day. The philosophy is that dieters would be more consistent rotating foods, as opposed to eating the same food at the same time every day of the week, for months.

The categories used here to break down exchanges are:

1. Mobility Movements to warm up.
2. Static Stretches
3. Foam Rolling Techniques
4. Low-level Neurological Activation Exercises
5. Lower Body Injury Prevention Exercises
6. Upper Body Injury Prevention Exercises
7. Plyometrics
8. Lower Body Strength-dominant Power Exercises
9. Lower Body Speed-dominant Power Exercises
10. Lower body Sport-specific Exercises
11. Upper body Sport-specific Exercises
12. Lateral Movements
13. Upper Body Strength-dominant Power Exercises
14. Upper Body Speed-dominant Power Exercises
15. Core

At minimum, each program should consist of at least these 5 components:

1. Warm-up (not required if warmed up from previous activity).
2. Injury prevention exercises.
3. Power development, broken down into 2 distinct methodologies:
    a. One or more heavier "functional" lifts to increase force production (Lower Body Strength-dominant Power Exercises), and
    b. One or more lighter, faster movements (Lower Body Speed-dominant Power Exercises) to promote more speed in the body and specificity in movement.
4. Individual Deficiency Training Exercises, for example, doing hip abduction exercises to strengthen the glutes if strength is a limiting factor in throwing high kicks, or med ball rotational throwing to help increase speed in rotating the trunk if that trait is lagging.
5. Core stabilization.

For a brief understanding of the distinction in power developmental exercises, examples of more functional /strength-dominant lifts can include all types of squats, trap bar deadlifts, all variations of cleans (like power cleans, hang cleans, cleans from blocks, clean pulls, clean pulls from blocks, etc.), lunges, and split squats. Faster, speed-dominant movements are not limited to the following, but might include resisted cord lateral hops, resisted cord blitzing, plyometrics of all kinds, squat jumps, step up jumps, split squat jumps, etc.

So therefore, a sample 45-minute two-day per week program for a developmental athlete with some time restrictions may look like this:

FIGURE 35:

	Day 1	S	R	%	W	
A	WARM UP	Not needed - coming from practice				
B	INJURY PREVENTION:					
	TUBING ANKLE DORSI FLEXION	1	10			
	TUBING ANKLE PLANTAR FLEXION	1	10			
	TUBING CLOCKWISE CIRCLES	1	10			
	TUBING COUNTERCLOCKWISE CIRCLES	1	10			
	TUBING INTERNAL SHOULDER ROTATIONS	1	10			
	TUBING EXTERNAL SHOULDER ROTATIONS	1	10			
C	FRONT SQUAT	1	5	50%	50	** BASED OFF OF 100 POUND MAX
		1	5	65%	65	** BASED OFF OF 100 POUND MAX
		1	5	75%	75	** BASED OFF OF 100 POUND MAX
D	CIRCUIT:					
	SPLIT SQUAT JUMPS	3	8			
	RESISTED CORD LATERAL HOPS	3	8			
	INVERTED ROW	3	8			
	MED BALL PUNCH PASS	3	8			

E	CIRCUIT:					
	LEFT SIDE PLANK	2	30 S			
	RIGHT SLIDE PLANK	2	30 S			
	LEFT SIDE BIRD DOG HOLD	2	30 S			
	RIGHT SIDE BIRD DOG HOLD	2	30 S			
	LEFT LEG MODIFIED HOLLOW BODY HOLD	2	30 S			
	RIGHT LEG MODIFIED HOLLOW BODY HOLD	2	30 S			

FIGURE 36:

Day 2		Week 1				
		S	R	%	W	
A	WARM UP	Not needed - coming from practice				
B	INJURY PREVENTION:					
	STANDING SCAPTION	1	10			
	SUPINE SCAPTION	1	10			
	PRONE INCLINE LATERAL RAISE	1	10			
	PLATE CIRCLES	1	10			
	TIB BAR FLEXION	1	10			
	UNSTABLE SURFACE BALANCING	1	10			
C	REAR FOOT ELEVATED SPLIT SQUAT	1	8			** Warm up weight
		1	8			** Pretty heavy
		1	8			** Heavy
D	CIRCUIT:					
	RESISTED CORD BLITZ	4	8			
	DUMBBELL SQUAT JUMPS	4	8			
	BENT OVER DUMBBELL ROW	4	8			
	STANDING HIGH SIDE KICKS	4	8			** Use ankle weights, kicks must be slow
E	CIRCUIT:					
	BACK EXTENSION HOLD	2	30 S			
	FEET ON BENCH RIGHT SLIDE PLANK	2	30 S			
	FEET ON BENCH LEFT SLIDE PLANK	2	30 S			
	SWISS BALL HOLLOW BODY HOLD	2	30 S			

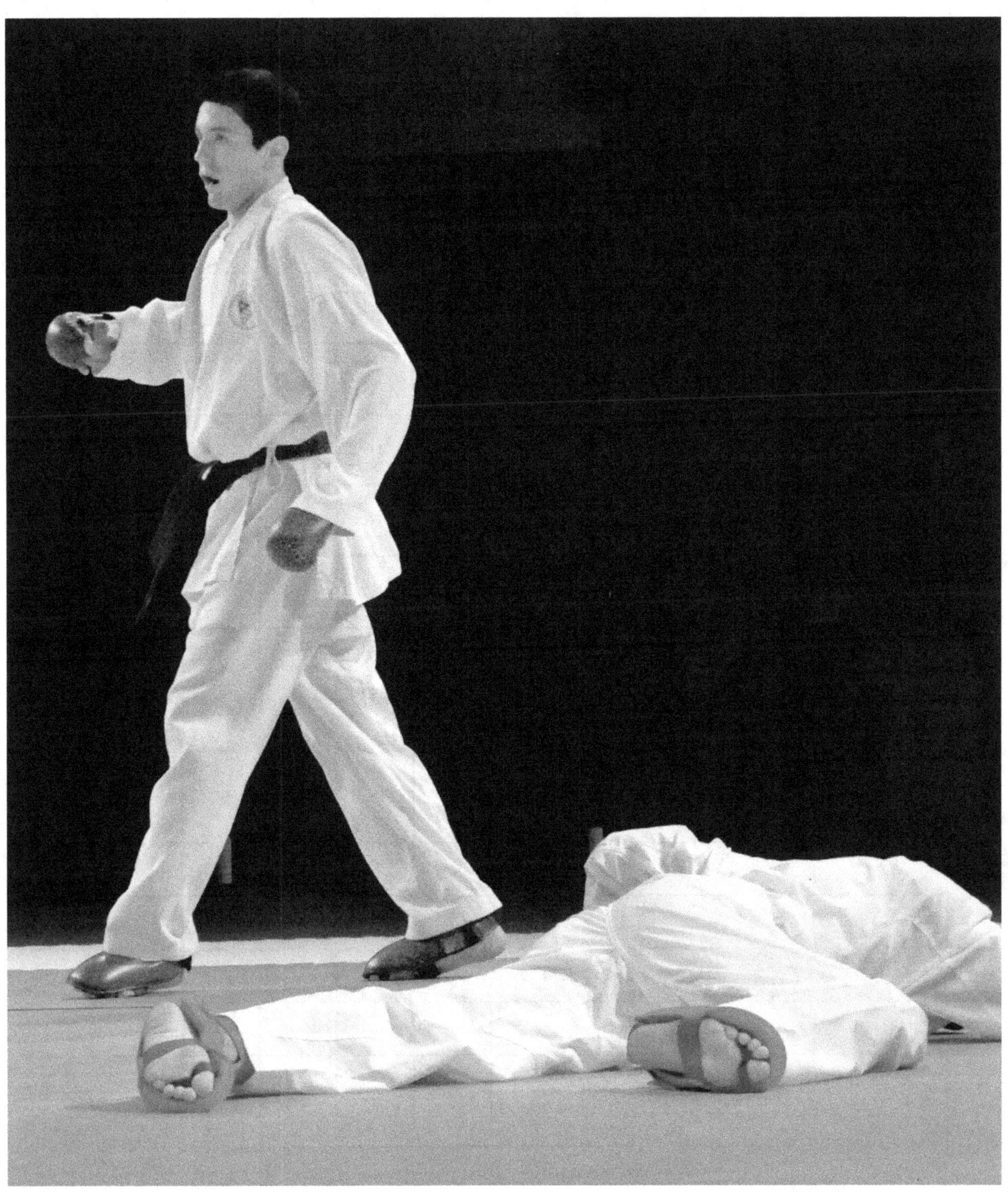

Justifications for inclusion of the chosen exercises in the program are listed in the note's column below.

FIGURE 37:

	Day 1	S	R	%	W	
A	**WARM UP**	Not needed - coming from practice				
B	**INJURY PREVENTION:**					
	TUBING ANKLE DORSI FLEXION	1	10			LOWER BODY INJURY PREVENTION
	TUBING ANKLE PLANTAR FLEXION	1	10			LOWER BODY INJURY PREVENTION
	TUBING CLOCKWISE CIRCLES	1	10			LOWER BODY INJURY PREVENTION
	TUBING COUNTER- CLOCKWISE CIRCLES	1	10			LOWER BODY INJURY PREVENTION
	TUBING INTERNAL SHOULDER ROTATIONS	1	10			UPPER BODY INJURY PREVENTION
	TUBING EXTERNAL SHOULDER ROTATIONS	1	10			UPPER BODY INJURY PREVENTION
C	**FRONT SQUAT**	1	5	50%	50	LOWER BODY STRENGTH-DOMINANT POWER EXERCISE
		1	5	65%	65	
		1	5	75%	75	
D	**CIRCUIT:**					
	SPLIT SQUAT JUMPS	3	8			LOWER BODY SPEED-DOMINANT POWER EXERCISE

	RESISTED CORD LATERAL HOPS	3	8			LOWER BODY SPEED-DOMINANT POWER EXERCISE/ LATERAL MOVEMENT/ SPORT-SPECIFIC
	INVERTED ROW	3	8			UPPER BODY STRENGTH-DOMINANT POWER EXERCISE/INJURY PREVENTION
	MED BALL PUNCH PASS	3	8			UPPER BODY SPEED-DOMINANT POWER EXERCISE/SPORT-SPECIFIC
E	**CIRCUIT:**					
	LEFT SIDE PLANK	2	30 S			CORE
	RIGHT SLIDE PLANK	2	30 S			CORE
	LEFT SIDE BIRD DOG HOLD	2	30 S			CORE
	RIGHT SIDE BIRD DOG HOLD	2	30 S			CORE
	LEFT LEG MODIFIED HOLLOW BODY HOLD	2	30 S			CORE
	RIGHT LEG MODIFIED HOLLOW BODY HOLD	2	30 S			CORE

Day 2		Week 1			
		S	**R**	**%**	**W**	
A	**WARM UP**	Not needed - coming from practice				
B	**INJURY PREVENTION:**					
	STANDING SCAPTION	1	10			UPPER BODY INJURY PREVENTION
	SUPINE SCAPTION	1	10			UPPER BODY INJURY PREVENTION
	PRONE INCLINE LATERAL RAISE	1	10			UPPER BODY INJURY PREVENTION
	PLATE CIRCLES	1	10			UPPER BODY INJURY PREVENTION
	TIB BAR FLEXION	1	10			LOWER BODY INJURY PREVENTION
	UNSTABLE SURFACE BALANCING	1	10			LOWER BODY INJURY PREVENTION
C	**REAR FOOT ELEVATED SPLIT SQUAT**	1	8			LOWER BODY STRENGTH-DOMINANT POWER EXERCISE
		1	8			
		1	8			
D	**CIRCUIT:**					
	RESISTED CORD BLITZ	4	8			LOWER BODY SPEED-DOMINANT POWER EXERCISE/ SPORT-SPECIFIC
	DUMBBELL SQUAT JUMPS	4	8			LOWER BODY SPEED-DOMINANT POWER EXERCISE
	BENT OVER DUMBBELL ROW	4	8			UPPER BODY STRENGTH-DOMINANT POWER EXERCISE/INJURY PREVENTION

						SPORTS-SPECIFIC/ DEFIENCY-SPECIFIC
	STANDING HIGH SIDE KICKS	4	8			
E	**CIRCUIT:**					
	BACK EXTENSION HOLD	2	30 S			CORE
	FEET ON BENCH RIGHT SLIDE PLANK	2	30 S			CORE
	FEET ON BENCH LEFT SLIDE PLANK	2	30 S			CORE
	SWISS BALL HOLLOW BODY HOLD	2	30 S			CORE

This is not to say that everyone should be on the aforementioned program. That was a hypothetical example of a pretty easy, but still very effective program. A variation for a more recreational-based athlete with even greater time restrictions might be condensed into a program that looks more like this. Once again, the notes column explains the reasoning for the prescription of the exercise.

FIGURE 39:

	Day 1	Week 1				
		S	**R**	**%**	**W**	
A	**WARM UP**	Not needed - coming from practice				
B	**CIRCUIT:**					
	INVERTED ROW	2	8			UPPER BODY STRENGTH-DOMINANT POWER EXERCISE/INJURY PREVENTION
	DUMBBELL SQUAT JUMPS	2	8			LOWER BODY SPEED-DOMINANT POWER EXERCISE
	PLANK ON SWISS BALL	2	45s			CORE
	SPLIT SQUAT JUMPS	2	8			LOWER BODY SPEED-DOMINANT POWER EXERCISE
	DUMBBELL BENCH PRESS	2	8			UPPER BODY STRENGTH-DOMINANT POWER EXERCISE
	RESISTED CORD LATERAL HOPS	2	8			LOWER BODY SPEED-DOMINANT POWER EXERCISE/ LATERAL MOVEMENT/ SPORTS-SPECIFIC
	HIGH HOOK KICKS	2	8			SPORTS-SPECIFIC/ DEFIENCY-SPECIFIC
	HIGH ROUNDHOUSE KICKS	2	8			SPORTS-SPECIFIC/ DEFIENCY-SPECIFIC

FIGURE 40:

	Day 2	S	R	%	W	
A	**WARM UP**	Not needed - coming from practice				
B	**CIRCUIT:**					
	RESISTED CORD BLITZ	3	8			LOWER BODY SPEED-DOMINANT POWER EXERCISE/SPORT-SPECIFIC
	BENT OVER DUMBBELL ROW	3	8			UPPER BODY STRENGTH-DOMINANT POWER EXERCISE/INJURY PREVENTION
	SPLIT SQUAT JUMPS	3	8			LOWER BODY SPEED-DOMINANT POWER EXERCISE
	LEFT AND RIGHT-SIDE PLANK	3	30 S			CORE
	MED BALL PUNCH PASS	3	8			UPPER BODY SPEED-DOMINANT POWER EXERCISE/SPORT-SPECIFIC
	BOSU BALL FRONT FOOT ELEVATED SPLIT SQUAT	3	8			LOWER BODY SPORTS-SPECIFIC POWER EXERCISE/INJURY PREVENTION
	WEIGHTED BOSU BALL PUSH-UP	3	max			UPPER BODY SPORTS-SPECIFIC POWER EXERCISE/INJURY PREVENTION
	ALT. HIGH HOOK + ROUNDHOUSE KICKS	3	8			SPORTS-SPECIFIC/DEFIENCY-SPECIFIC

Obviously, this is really basic, and hopefully you've noticed some things missing that would make it much better, like more injury prevention, but this program, despite its limitations, can still create positive changes for a karateka. In fact, even two sets of this circuit can be extremely beneficial, compared to not training at all. Remember, something is better than nothing.

The purpose of this next section is to provide examples for the exchange lists, to serve as a tentative guide for your program construction. Please note, these are not fully comprehensive.

Indeed, they are very long and list hundreds of choices, but other choices can also work. It was our desire to afford readers to ability to create meaningful programs, not to list all exercises, including less-productive movements. They are arranged in no special order, so the first exercise listed is not necessarily more useful than the ones below it. Lastly, some exercises may not be interchangeable with others, even though they fall in the same category. For instance, internal rotations and external rotations do opposite functions and an athlete with over developed internal rotators should choose exercises to promote strength in the external rotators and balance in the shoulder, and not just do more internal rotation work. This is commonsensical.

FIGURE 41:

1. MOBILITY MOVEMENTS (All are dynamic movements, typically done over 10-15 meters)
    - Walking Forward, Forward Arm Circles
    - Walking Forward, Backward Arm Circles
    - Knee to Chest Walk
    - Leg Cradles
    - Quads
    - Backwards hamstring
    - Quad with RDL
    - Lateral Groin – both directions
    - Cross Over Toe Touch
    - Forward Kicks
    - Twisting Lunges
    - Kick skips
    - Open the Gate Walk
    - Close the Gate Walk
    - Walking Backwards, Backwards Straight Leg Kicks
    - Side Shuffle Side Leg Raise
    - Side shuffle Ground Swoop
    - Lateral Groin Lunge with Crossover Lunge
    - Side Shuffle Curtsy Lunge
    - Walking Lunge into "World's Greatest Stretch"
    - Straight Leg Lunge Walk into Alternating Kicks

2. STATIC STRETCHES (some are named with yoga terminology)

- Standing Calf
- Push-up Position Calf
- Child's Pose
- Cobra Pose
- Downward dog
- Left Leg Forward Pigeon Pose
- Right Leg Forward Pigeon Pose
- Left Leg half Kneeling Hip Flexor
- Right Leg half Kneeling Hip Flexor
- Left Leg half Kneeling Hip Flexor with Quad
- Right Leg half Kneeling Hip Flexor with Quad
- Butterfly pulling on Feet
- Butterfly Elbows on Knees Pushing Down
- Left Side Lying Quad
- Right Side Lying Quad

3. FOAM ROLLING TECHNIQUES

- Left Calf
- Right Calf
- Left Hamstring
- Right Hamstring
- Left Glute
- Right Glute
- Left IT band
- Right IT band
- Left Quad
- Right Quad
- Left Groin
- Right Groin

4. LOW-LEVEL NEURAL WARM-UPS

- LADDER DRILLS
  - ◊ Running 1 per box
  - ◊ Running 2 per box
  - ◊ Running 3 per box
  - ◊ In, In, Out
  - ◊ In, In, Out Backwards
  - ◊ In, In, Out, Out
  - ◊ In, In, Out, Out Backwards
  - ◊ High Knee Run
  - ◊ Short Ali Shuffle
  - ◊ Long Ali Shuffle
  - ◊ Crossover In, Out, Out
  - ◊ Backwards Crossover In, Out, Out
  - ◊ 2-foot hopscotch
  - ◊ Backwards Hopscotch
  - ◊ Shuffle every other box
  - ◊ In, In, Out every other box
  - ◊ In, In, Out, Out every other box
  - ◊ Butt Kick Run
  - ◊ Sideways Hopscotch
  - ◊ Single Leg Hops

- JUMP ROPE
  - ◊ 2-feet jump
  - ◊ Running in Place
  - ◊ Side to Side Hops (alpine ski)
  - ◊ Ali Shuffle (cross country ski)
  - ◊ Forward to Backward Hops
  - ◊ Alternating Side to Side and Forward to Backwards Hops
  - ◊ Single Leg Jump: Side to Side Hops (alpine ski)
  - ◊ Single Leg Jump: Forward to Backward Hops
  - ◊ Single Leg Jump: Alternating Side to Side and Forward to Backwards Hops
  - ◊ One Left, One Right, Two Left, 2 Right, etc.
  - ◊ Criss Cross
  - ◊ Double Leg Any Shape (triangle, square, rectangle, box, star)
- LINE HOPS
  - ◊ 2 Feet Side to side
  - ◊ Double Leg Forward to Backward Hops
  - ◊ Ali Shuffle (cross country ski)
  - ◊ Alternating Side to Side and Forward to Backwards Hops
  - ◊ Single Leg Hop: Side to Side Hops (alpine ski)
  - ◊ Single Leg Hop: Forward to Backward Hops
  - ◊ Single Leg Hop: Alternating Side to Side and Forward to Backwards Hops
  - ◊ Double Leg Any Shape (triangle, square, rectangle, box, star)
  - ◊ Single Leg Any Shape (triangle, square, rectangle, box, star)
  - ◊ Double Leg Forward to Backward Hops turning 90 Degrees
  - ◊ Single Leg Forward to Backward Hops turning 90 Degrees

- LOW BOX/AEROBICS STEP PATTERNS
  - ◊ Double Leg Forward to Backward Hops
  - ◊ Double Leg Side to Side Hops
  - ◊ One Up, Two Down
  - ◊ Ali Shuffle (cross country ski)
  - ◊ Ali Shuffle Double Touches
  - ◊ Ali Shuffle Alternating Single and Double Touches
  - ◊ Side to Side Double Touches
  - ◊ Side to Side Alternating Single and Double Touches
  - ◊ Side to Side Two Up One Down
- DOT DRILL PAD
  - ◊ Double Leg Side to Side Hops
  - ◊ Double Leg Forward to Backward Hops
  - ◊ Double Leg Diagonal Hops
  - ◊ Double Leg Any Shape (triangle, square, rectangle, box, star)
  - ◊ Ali Shuffle (cross country ski)
  - ◊ Single Leg Jump: Forward to Backward Hops
  - ◊ Single Leg Jump: Side to Side Hops (alpine ski)
  - ◊ Single Leg Jump: Alternating Side to Side and Forward to Backwards Hops
  - ◊ Single Leg Any Shape (triangle, square, rectangle, box, star)
  - ◊ Double Leg Forward to Backward Hops turning 90 Degree
  - ◊ Single Leg Forward to Backward Hops turning 90 Degree
  - ◊ Double Leg Touch All Exterior Dots Returning to Cente
  - ◊ Single Leg Touch All Exterior Dots Returning to Center
  - ◊ Forward and Backward Hopscotch Alternating One Foot on Center

- MINI HURDLES
    ◊ Jogging
    ◊ Unilateral High knee
    ◊ Unilateral Butt Kick
    ◊ Shuffling
    ◊ Double Leg Forward Hops
    ◊ Double Leg 180 Degree Hops
    ◊ Single Leg Forward Hops
    ◊ Single Leg Hops Moving Medial
    ◊ Single Leg Hops Moving Lateral
    ◊ Single Leg Forward Hops with Double Hop in Place
    ◊ Single Leg Hops Moving Medial with Double Hop in Place
    ◊ Single Leg Hops Moving Lateral with Double Hop in Place

5. LOWER BODY INJURY PREVENTION EXERCISES

- Marching on Heels (small steps, fast tempo, toes high)
- Marching on Toes
- Small Choppy High Knees (toes pointed in slightly)
- Small Choppy High Knees (toes pointed out slightly)
- Ankling
- Tibialis Anterior Bar Flexions
- Tibialis Anterior Tubing Flexions
- Tibialis Anterior Isometric Hold
- Tibialis Anterior Clockwise Circles
- Tibialis Anterior Counter-clockwise Circles
- Eccentric-dominant Heel Raises
- Single Leg Heel Raise
- Single Leg Heel Raise with Toes Pointed In
- Single Leg Heel Raise with Toes Pointed Out
- Tubing Dorsi Flexions
- Tubing Plantar Flexions
- Tubing Clockwise Circles
- Tubing Counter-clockwise Circles
- Unstable Surface Balancing (Bosu Ball, Airex Pad, Dyna Disc, etc.)
- Depth Drops
- Single Leg Depth Drops
- Single Leg Forward Hop Sticking the Landing in a Power Position
- Single Leg Sideways Hop Sticking the Landing in a Power Position
- Single Leg Backwards Hop Sticking the Landing in the Power Position
- Single Leg Backwards to Forward Hops Sticking Only the Forward Hop
- Single Leg Forward to Backward Hops Sticking Only the Backward Hop

6. UPPER BODY INJURY PREVENTION EXERCISES

- Supine Internal Rotation Stretch
- Suping External Rotation Stretch
- Side Lying Internal Rotation
- Side Lying External Rotation
- Tubing Internal Rotation
- Tubing External Rotation
- Prone Front Raise
- Prone Lateral Raise
- Prone Y's
- Bent Over Front Raise
- Bent Over Lateral Raise
- Bent Over Shoulder Extension
- Bent Over Y's
- Prone Incline Front Raise
- Prone Incline Lateral Raise
- Prone Incline Shoulder Extension
- Prone Incline Y's
- Scaptions
- Supine Scaptions
- Plate Circles
- Single Arm Dumbbell Pullover
- Band Pull Apart
- Inverted Row

7. PLYOMETRICS

- All Line Hops
- All Jump Rope Drills
- All Dot Drill Hops
- Power Skip for Height
- Power Skip for Distance
- Power Skip Uphill for Height
- Power Skip Uphill for Distance
- Bounding for Height
- Bounding for Distance
- Bounding Uphill for Height
- Bounding Uphill for Distance
- Double Leg Up, Up, Out Jump
- Double Leg Out, Out, Up Jump
- Double Leg Up, Out, Up Jump
- Repeat Box Jumps
- Double Leg Hurdle Hops Going Straight
- Double Leg Hurdle Hops Going Right or Left
- Double Leg Hurdle Hops in a Square
- Double 180 Degree Hurdle Hops
- Single Leg Up, Up, Out Jump
- Single Leg Out, Out, Up Jump
- Single Leg Up, Out, Up Jump
- Single Leg Hurdle Hops Going Straight
- Single Leg Hurdle Hops Going Right or Left
- Single Leg Hurdle Hops in a Square
- Single 180 Degree Hurdle Hops

8. STRENGTH-DOMINANT POWER EXERCISES

- Squat
- Narrow Stance Squat
- Pause Squat
- Front Squat
- Goblet Squat
- Squat Jumps (Heavy)
- Trap Bar Deadlift
- Rear Foot Elevated Split Squat
- Front Foot Elevated Split Squat
- Goblet Split Squat
- Front Rack Split Squat
- Lunges
- Walking Lunge
- Backwards Lunge
- Power Clean
- Hang Clean
- Clean from Blocks
- Dumbbell Cleans
- Clean Grip Snatch
- Clean Pull
- Snatch Pull
- Snatch
- Curtsy Lunge
- Cross Over Step-up
- Step-up
- Single Leg Squat
- Goblet Single Leg Squat
- Overhead Squat
- Good Morning

9. SPEED-DOMINANT POWER EXERCISES

- Step-up Jump
- Walking Lunge Jump
- Dumbbell Squat Jump (Light)
- Split Squat Jump
- Dumbbell Swings
- Kettle Bell Swings
- Rear Foot Elevated Split Squat Jumps
- Side Step-up Jumps
- Slide Board
- Resisted Sled Running
- Resisted Sled Pushing
- Resisted Cord Sprinting
- Assisted Cord Sprinting
- Resisted Cord Shuffling
- Rear Foot Elevated Split Squat Jumps

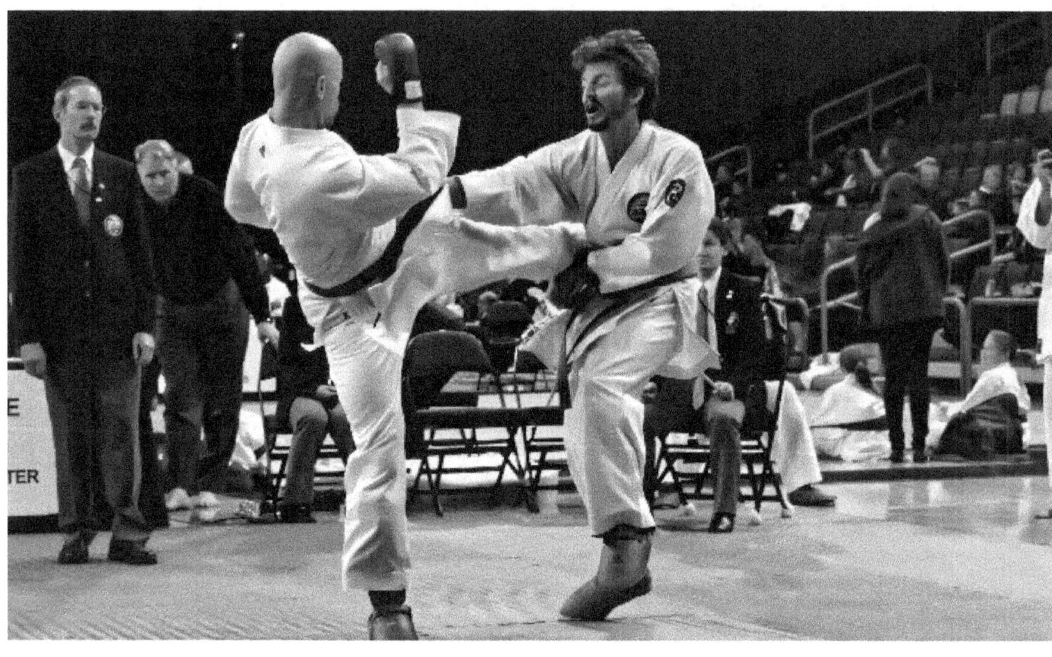

10. SPORT-SPECIFIC LOWER BODY

- Resisted Cord Blitz
- Resisted Cord Retreat
- Resisted Cord Straight Retreat and Angle
- Slow Front Kicks with Ankle Weights
- Slow Roundhouse Kicks with Ankle Weights
- Slow Side Kicks with Ankle Weights
- Slow Hook Kicks with Ankle Weights
- Resisted Cord Roundhouse Kick
- Resisted Cord Front Kick
- Resisted Cord Side Kick
- Resisted Cord Hook Kick
- All Kicks with Ankle Weight Over Table
- All Kicks with Isometric Starting Position Off Box
- Ankle Weight Adduction
- Side Lying Ankle Weight Adduction
- Band Resisted Punching
- Band Assisted Punching
- Medicine Ball Punch Pass

11. SPORT-SPECIFIC UPPER BODY

- Resisted Cord Punch
- Assisted Cord Punch
- Medicine Ball Punch Passes
- Medicine Ball Chest Passes

12. LATERAL MOVEMENT

- Lateral Squat
- Lateral Lunge
- Resisted Cord Shuffle
- Resisted Cord Lateral Hops
- Rope Hops
- Slide Board
- Resisted Cord Shuffle and Med Ball Punch Pass

13. UPPER BODY STRENGTH-DOMINANT POWER EXERCISES

- Dumbbell Bench Press
- Alternate Arm Dumbbell Bench Press
- Bent Over Dumbbell Row
- Inverted Row
- Close Grip Push-up
- Close Grip Push-up on Bosu Ball
- Weighted Chin-up
- Weighted Pull-up

14. UPPER BODY SPEED-DOMINANT POWER EXERCISES

- Medicine Ball Chest Pass
- Medicine Ball Punch Pass
- Resisted Cord Punch
- Assisted Cord Punch
- Clapping Push-ups

15. CORE

- Superman's
- Superman Hold on Back Extension Bench
- Plank
- Side Plank on Hand
- Side Plank on Forearm
- Side Plank with Hip Abduction Raises
- Side Plank with Hip Abduction Hold
- Hollow Body Holds
- One Leg Bent Hollow Body Hold
- Planks Flexing Legs to Opposite Arm
- Inverted Planks
- Inverted Plank with One Leg Up
- Planks Lifting One Arm
- Planks Lifting one Leg
- Flutter Kicks Lying Supine
- Planks with Hands on Ball, Feet on Bench
- Planks with Hands on Bench, Feet on Ball
- Planks with Hands on Ball, Feet on Ground
- Planks with Hands on Ground, Feet on Ball
- Forearm Rollout on Ball
- Chin in Hands, Elbows on Ground Plank
- Ball Planks on forearms
- Resisted Cord Punches
- Resisted Cord Rotations
- Medicine Ball Rotational Throws
- Medicine Ball Punch Pass

Now we have choices, lots of choices. It's time to assign a time to each of the workout priorities and create the daily template. For example, a karateka coming from practice, as we have seen before, would not be wise to waste 10-15 minutes on a warm-up, because they are already warmed up. Likewise, a power-deficient athlete may need additional time on more strength-dominant power exercises, so more time should be allotted there. The following examples for a novice and intermediate trainee show some differing protocols, and the structure that determines the daily format.

FIGURE 42:

Sample Template: Novice 2x week 1 hour Program		
PERIOD	TIME	OBJECTIVES
1	10 Minutes	Mobilities/Stretching
2	10 Minutes	Warm-up Injury Prevention
3	10 Minutes	Strength-Dominant Power Lower Body Strength-Dominant Power Upper Body
4	20 Minutes	Power/Sports Specific/Deficiencies
5	10 Minutes	Core

In this format, the athlete needs ample warm-up time (10 minutes). Injury prevention receives 10 minutes of the hour as well. Lower body and upper body strength-dominant exercises are supersetted (alternated) to make the work-out as efficient as possible timewise. Additional development is accomplished in a 20-minute period allotted to power development, sport-specific movements, and individual deficiencies. The last ten minutes are devoted to core stabilization.

Written out in a one-week format, a 2-time per week protocol might look like this:

FIGURE 43:

Sample Template: Novice 2x week 1 hour Program				Week 1				Notes
PERIOD	TIME	OBJECTIVES	EXERCISE	S	R	%	W	
1	10 min	**Mobilities/Stretching**	**Walking Forward, Forward Arm Circles**	1	10M			
			Walking Forward, Backward Arm Circles	1	10M			
			Knee to Chest Walk	1	10M			
			Leg Cradles	1	10M			
			Quads	1	10M			
			Backwards hamstring	1	10M			
			Quad with RDL	1	10M			
			Lateral Groin – both directions	1	10M			

			Cross Over Toe Touch	1	10M			
			Forward Kicks	1	10M			
			Twisting Lunges	1	10M			
			Kick skips	1	10M			
			Open the Gate Walk	1	10M			
			Close the Gate Walk	1	10M			
2	10 min	Warm-up /Injury Prevention	Low Box Ali Shuffle	2	10			Circuit
			Tubing External Rotation	2	10			Circuit
			Tubing Ankle Dorsi Flexion	2	10			Circuit
			Bent Over Lateral Raise	2	10			Circuit
			Jump Rope Side to Side	2	10			Circuit
			Unstable Surface Balancing	2	30 Sec			Circuit
3	10 min	Strength-Dominant Power Lower Body	Single Leg Split Squat	3	5			Superset
		Strength-Dominant Power Upper Body	Close Grip Push-up on Bosu Ball	3	15			Superset
4	20 min	Power/Sports Specific/ Deficiencies	Dumbbell Squat Jumps	2	8			Circuit
			Inverted Row	2	8			Circuit
			Slide Board	2	20			Circuit
			Medicine Ball Punch Pass	2	8			Circuit
5	10 min	Core	Plank: Hands on Ball, Feet on Bench	2	30 Sec			Circuit
			Left Side Plank on Hand	2	30 Sec			Circuit
			Right Side Plank on Hand	2	30 Sec			Circuit
			Superman Hold on Back Extension Machine	2	30 Sec			Circuit

FIGURE 44:

Sample Template 2: Novice 2x week 1 hour Program				Week 1				Notes
PERIOD	TIME	OBJECTIVES	EXERCISE	S	R	%	W	
1	10 min	Mobilities/Stretching	Standing Calf	1	30 Sec			
			Push-up Position Calf	1	30 Sec			
			Child's Pose	1	30 Sec			
			Cobra Pose	1	30 Sec			
			Downward dog	1	30 Sec			
			Left Leg Forward Pigeon Pose	1	30 Sec			
			Right Leg Forward Pigeon Pose	1	30 Sec			
			Left Leg half Kneeling Hip Flexor	1	30 Sec			
			Right Leg half Kneeling Hip Flexor	1	30 Sec			
			Left Leg half Kneeling Hip Flexor with Quad	1	30 Sec			
			Right Leg half Kneeling Hip Flexor with Quad	1	30 Sec			
			Butterfly pulling on Feet	1	30 Sec			
			Butterfly Elbows on Knees Pushing Down	1	30 Sec			
			Left Side Lying Quad	1	30 Sec			
			Right Side Lying Quad	1	30 Sec			
2	10 min	Warm-up Injury Prevention	Ladder: In, In, Out	2				Circuit
			Tubing Pull Aparts	2	10			Circuit
			Tubing Clockwise and Counterclockwise Ankle Circles	2	10			Circuit
			Single Arm Dumbbell Pullover	2	10			Circuit
			Depth Drops	2	5			Circuit
			Plate Circles	2	10/e			Circuit

3	10 min	Strength-Dominant Power Lower Body	Goblet Squat	3	5			Superset
		Strength-Dominant Power Upper Body	Alternate Arm Dumbbell Bench Press	3	8/e			Superset
4	20 min	Power/Sport- Specific/ Deficiencies	Repeat Box Hops	2	8			Circuit
			Bent Over Dumbbell Rows	2	8			Circuit
			Curtsy Lunge	2	8			Circuit
			Rotational Medicine Ball Throw	2	8			Circuit
5	10 min	Core	Left Leg Bent Hollow Body Hold	2	30 Sec			Circuit
			Right Leg Bent Hollow Body Hold	2	30 Sec			Circuit
			Left Plank on Forearm	2	30 Sec			Circuit
			Right Plank on Forearm	2	30 Sec			Circuit
			Left Leg, Right Arm Bird Dog	2	30 Sec			Circuit
			Right Leg, Left Arm Bird Dog	2	30 Sec			Circuit

Another way a 2x per week can be formatted can look like this. This is an example for an intermediate trainee.

FIGURE 45:

Sample Template: Intermediate 2x week 1 hour Program		
PERIOD	TIME	OBJECTIVES
1	15 Minutes	Warm-up/Mobility
2	15 Minutes	Lower Body Strength-Dominant Power Lower Body Speed-Dominant Power
3	15 Minutes	Upper Body Strength-Dominant Power Upper Body Speed-Dominant Power
4	15 Minutes	Core/Injury Prevention/Power

Examples of the two days can be:

FIGURE 46:

Sample Template: Intermediate 2x week 1 hour Program				Week 1				Notes
PERIOD	**TIME**	**OBJECTIVES**	**EXERCISE**	**S**	**R**	**%**	**W**	
1	15 min	**Warm-up/Mobility**	**Calf Stretch**	2	30 Sec			Circuit
			Double Leg Jump Rope	2	30 Sec			Circuit
			Quad Walk with RDL	2	10M			Circuit
			Mini Hurdle Shuffling Right and Left	2	10M			Circuit
			Straight Leg Lunge with Kicks	2	10M			Circuit
			Ali Shuffle Jump Rope	2	30 Sec			Circuit
			Plate Circles	2	10/E			Circuit
			Side Shuffle Side Leg Raise	2	10M			Circuit
2	15 min	**Lower Body Strength-Dominant Power**	**Squat**	4	5			Superset
		Lower Body Speed-Dominant Power	**Forward Hurdle Hops**	4	5			Superset
3	15 min	**Upper Body Strength-Dominant Power**	**Dumbbell Bench Press**	4	5			Superset
		Upper Body Speed-Dominant Power	**Medicine Ball Chest Pass**	4	5			Superset
4	15 min	**Core/Injury Prevention/ Power**	**Resisted Cord Blitz**	2	5			Circuit
			Hollow Body Hold	2	30 Sec			Circuit
			Resisted Cord Lateral Hops	2	8/e			Circuit
			Weighted Chin-up	2	5			Circuit
			Hook Kick off Box	2	8/e		ankle	Circuit

FIGURE 47:

Sample Template 2: Intermediate 2x week 1 hour Program				Week 1				Notes
PERIOD	**TIME**	**OBJECTIVES**	**EXERCISE**	**S**	**R**	**%**	**W**	
1	15 min	Warm-up/Mobility	Calf Stretch	2	30 Sec			Circuit
			Ladder: Cross Over in, out, out	2				Circuit
			Tubing Pull Apart	2	10			Circuit
			Ladder Ali Shuffle	2				Circuit
			Supine Scaption	2	10			Circuit
			Lateral Groin with Crossover Lunge	2	20M			Circuit
			Quad with RDL	2	20 M			Circuit
			Straight Leg Lunge with Kick	2	20 M			Circuit
2	15 min	Lower Body Strength-Dominant Power	Hang Clean	4	5			Superset
		Lower Body Speed-Dominant Power	Tuck Jumps	4	5			Superset
3	15 min	Upper Body Strength-Dominant Power	Alternate Arm Dumbbell Bench Press	4	5			Superset
		Upper Body Speed-Dominant Power	Medicine Ball Punch Pass	4	5			Superset
4	15 min	Core/Injury Prevention/Power	Resisted Cord Blitz	2	5			Circuit
			Plank on Swiss Ball	2	60			Circuit
			Weighted Roundhouse Kick	2	8/e		ankle	Circuit
			Weighted Chin-up	2	5			Circuit
			Weighted Side Kick	2	8/e		ankle	Circuit

PLANNING THE MONTHLY FORMAT

Incorporating the principles we learned earlier, the monthly format can be finalized for our novice lifter this way. Notice how the first week is the lowest in volume, and how there is increasing difficulty in weeks two and three. Interestingly, week four is not any less intense because the load should actually increase (overload principle), but the volume decreases a little bit. This is to train efficiently and safely and to ensure that we don't overtrain. The combination of lower volume with increased fitness and familiarity helps the total week to be less taxing. This is often referred to as a "lighter week" or "de-load week."

FIGURE 48:

	Day 1	Week 1				Week 2				Week 3				Week 4				Notes
	EXERCISE	S	R	%	W	S	R	%	W	S	R	%	W	S	R	%	W	
A	Walking Forward, Forward Arm Circles	1	10M			1	10M			1	10M			1	10M			
	Walking Forward, Backward Arm Circles	1	10M			1	10M			1	10M			1	10M			
	Knee to Chest Walk	1	10M			1	10M			1	10M			1	10M			
	Leg Cradles	1	10M			1	10M			1	10M			1	10M			
	Quads	1	10M			1	10M			1	10M			1	10M			
	Backwards hamstring	1	10M			1	10M			1	10M			1	10M			
	Quad with RDL	1	10M			1	10M			1	10M			1	10M			
	Lateral Groin – both directions	1	10M			1	10M			1	10M			1	10M			
	Cross Over Toe Touch	1	10M			1	10M			1	10M			1	10M			
	Forward Kicks	1	10M			1	10M			1	10M			1	10M			
	Twisting Lunges	1	10M			1	10M			1	10M			1	10M			
	Kick skips	1	10M			1	10M			1	10M			1	10M			
	Open the Gate Walk	1	10M			1	10M			1	10M			1	10M			
	Close the Gate Walk	1	10M			1	10M			1	10M			1	10M			
B	Low Box Ali Shuffle	2	10			2	10			2	10			2	10			Circuit
	Tubing External Rotation	2	10			2	10			2	10			2	10			Circuit
	Tubing Ankle Dorsi Flexion	2	10			2	10			2	10			2	10			Circuit
	Bent Over Lateral Raise	2	10			2	10			2	10			2	10			Circuit
	Jump Rope Side to Side	2	10			2	10			2	10			2	10			Circuit

	Unstable Surface Balancing	2	30 Sec			2	30 Sec			2	30 Sec			2	30 Sec			Circuit
C	Single Leg Split Squat	3	5			4	7			4	8			4	5			Superset
	Close Grip Push-up on Bosu Ball	3	15			4	15			4	Max			4	Max			Superset
D	Dumbbell Squat Jumps	2	8			3	8			3	8			3	8			Circuit
	Inverted Row	2	8			3	10			3	Max			3	Max			Circuit
	Slide Board	2	20			3	20			3	20			3	20			Circuit
	Medicine Ball Punch Pass	2	8			3	8			3	8			3	8			Circuit
E	Plank: Hands on Ball Feet on Bench	2	30 Sec			2	45 Sec			2	60 Sec			2	45 Sec			Circuit
	Left Side Plank on Hand	2	30 Sec			2	45 Sec			2	60 Sec			2	45 Sec			Circuit
	Right Side Plank on Hand	2	30 Sec			2	45 Sec			2	60 Sec			2	45 Sec			Circuit
	Superman Hold on Back Extension Machine	2	30 Sec			2	45 Sec			2	60 Sec			2	45 Sec			Circuit

Day 2		Week 1				Week 2				Week 3				Week 4				Notes
	EXERCISE	S	R	%	W	S	R	%	W	S	R	%	W	S	R	%	W	
A	Standing Calf	1	30 Sec			1	30 Sec			1	30 Sec			1	30 Sec			
	Push-up Position Calf	1	30 Sec			1	30 Sec			1	30 Sec			1	30 Sec			
	Child's Pose	1	30 Sec			1	30 Sec			1	30 Sec			1	30 Sec			
	Cobra Pose	1	30 Sec			1	30 Sec			1	30 Sec			1	30 Sec			
	Downward dog	1	30 Sec			1	30 Sec			1	30 Sec			1	30 Sec			
	Left Leg Forward Pigeon Pose	1	30 Sec			1	30 Sec			1	30 Sec			1	30 Sec			
	Right Leg Forward Pigeon Pose	1	30 Sec			1	30 Sec			1	30 Sec			1	30 Sec			
	Left Leg half Kneeling Hip Flexor	1	30 Sec			1	30 Sec			1	30 Sec			1	30 Sec			
	Right Leg half Kneeling Hip Flexor	1	30 Sec			1	30 Sec			1	30 Sec			1	30 Sec			
	Left Leg half Kneeling Hip Flexor with Quad	1	30 Sec			1	30 Sec			1	30 Sec			1	30 Sec			
	Right Leg half Kneeling Hip Flexor with Quad	1	30 Sec			1	30 Sec			1	30 Sec			1	30 Sec			
	Butterfly pulling on Feet	1	30 Sec			1	30 Sec			1	30 Sec			1	30 Sec			
	Butterfly Elbows on Knees Pushing Down	1	30 Sec			1	30 Sec			1	30 Sec			1	30 Sec			
	Left Side Lying Quad	1	30 Sec			1	30 Sec			1	30 Sec			1	30 Sec			
	Right Side Lying Quad	1	30 Sec			1	30 Sec			1	30 Sec			1	30 Sec			
B	Ladder In, In, out	2				2				2				2				Circuit
	Tubing Pull Aparts	2	10			2	10			2	10			2	10			Circuit
	Tubing Clockwise/ Counterclockwise Ankle Circles	2	10			2	10			2	10			2	10			Circuit
	Single Arm Dumbbell Row	2	10			2	10			2	10			2	10			Circuit
	Depth Drops	2	5			2	5			2	5			2	5			Circuit
	Plate Circles	2	10 each			2	10 each			2	10 each			2	10 each			Circuit

C	Goblet Squat	3	5			4	5			4	8			4	5			Superset
	Alternate Arm Dumbbell Bench Press	3	8 each			4	8 each			4	10 each			4	8 each			Superset
D	Repeat Box Hops	2	8			3	8			3	10			2	8			Circuit
	Bent Over Dumbbell Rows	2	8			3	8			3	10			2	8			Circuit
	Curtsy Lunge	2	8			3	8			3	10			2	8			Circuit
	Rotational Medicine Ball Throw	2	8			3	8			3	10			2	8			Circuit
E	Left Leg Bent Hollow Body Hold	2	30 Sec			2	35 Sec			2	40 Sec			1	60 Sec			Circuit
	Right Leg Bent Hollow Body Hold	2	30 Sec			2	35 Sec			2	40 Sec			1	60 Sec			Circuit
	Left Plank on Forearm	2	30 Sec			2	35 Sec			2	40 Sec			1	60 Sec			Circuit
	Right Plank on Forearm	2	30 Sec			2	35 Sec			2	40 Sec			1	60 Sec			Circuit
	Left Leg, Right Arm Bird Dog	2	30 Sec			2	35 Sec			2	40 Sec			1	60 Sec			Circuit
	Right Leg, Left Arm Bird Dog	2	30 Sec			2	35 Sec			2	40 Sec			1	60 Sec			Circuit

The intermediate-experienced lifter's monthly format might now appear as follows. Like the novice lifter, this karateka has an introductory week in the cycle, followed by two harder weeks and a de-load week. Because this athlete has more training experience, he/she is prescribed sets of fewer reps on the heavier lifts, like squats, cleans and dumbbell bench presses.

FIGURE 50:

DAY 1		Week 1				Week 2				Week 3				Week 4				Notes
	EXERCISE	S	R	%	W	S	R	%	W	S	R	%	W	S	R	%	W	
A	Calf Stretch	2	30 Sec			2	30 Sec			2	30 Sec			2	30 Sec			Circuit
	Double Leg Jump Rope	2	30 Sec			2	30 Sec			2	30 Sec			2	30 Sec			Circuit
	Quad Walk with RDL	2	10M			2	10M			2	10M			2	10M			Circuit
	Mini Hurdle Shuffling Right and Left	2	10M			2	10M			2	10M			2	10M			Circuit
	Straight Leg Lunge with Kicks	2	10M			2	10M			2	10M			2	10M			Circuit
	Ali Shuffle Jump Rope	2	30 Sec			2	30 Sec			2	30 Sec			2	30 Sec			Circuit
	Plate Circles	2	10 Each			2	10 Each			2	10 Each			2	10 Each			Circuit
	Side Shuffle Side Leg Raise	2	10M			2	10M			2	10M			2	10M			Circuit
B	Squat	4	5			5	5			5	4			4	3			Superset
	Forward Hurdle Hops	4	5			5	5			5	5			4	5			Superset
C	Dumbbell Bench Press	4	5			5	5			5	5			4	5			Superset
	Medicine Ball Chest Pass	4	5			5	5			5	5			4	5			Superset
D	Resisted Cord Blitz	2	5			3	5			4	5			3	5			Circuit
	Hollow Body Hold	2	30 Sec			3	30 Sec			4	30 Sec			3	30 Sec			Circuit
	Resisted Cord Lateral Hops	2	8 Each			3	8 Each			4	8 Each			3	8 Each			Circuit
	Weighted Chin-up	2	5			3	5			4	5			3	5			Circuit
	Hook Kick off Box	2	8 Each		ankle	3	8 Each		ankle	4	8 Each		ankle	3	8 Each		ankle	Circuit

FIGURE 51:

	DAY 2	Week 1				Week 2				Week 3				Week 4				Notes
	EXERCISE	S	R	%	W	S	R	%	W	S	R	%	W	S	R	%	W	
A	Calf Stretch	2	30 Sec			2	30 Sec			2	30 Sec			2	30 Sec			Circuit
	Ladder: Cross Over in, out, out	2				2				2				2				Circuit
	Tubing Pull Apart	2	10			2	10			2	10			2	10			Circuit
	Ladder Ali Shuffle	2				2				2				2				Circuit
	Supine Scaptions	2	10			2	10			2	10			2	10			Circuit
	Lateral Groin with Crossover Lunge	2	20M			2	20M			2	20M			2	20M			Circuit
	Quad with RDL	2	20 M			2	20 M			2	20 M			2	20 M			Circuit
	Straight Leg Lunge with Kick	2	20 M			2	20 M			2	20 M			2	20 M			Circuit
B	Hang Clean	4	5			5	4			5	3			4	3			Superset
	Tuck Jumps	4	5			5	5			5	5			4	5			Superset
C	Alternate Arm Dumbbell Bench Press	4	5			5	5			5	5			4	5			Superset
	Medicine Ball Punch Pass	4	5			5	5			5	5			4	5			Superset
D	Resisted Cord Blitz	2	5			3	5			3	5			3	5			Circuit
	Plank on Swiss Ball	2	60			3	60			3	60			3	60			Circuit
	Weighted Roundhouse Kick	2	8 Each		ankle	3	8 Each		ankle	3	8 Each		ankle	3	8 Each		ankle	Circuit
	Weighted Chin-up	2	5			3	5			3	5			3	5			Circuit
	Weighted Side Kick	2	8 Each		ankle	3	8 Each		ankle	3	8 Each		ankle	3	8 Each		ankle	Circuit

FINAL THOUGHTS ON STRENGTH TRAINING PROGRAM DESIGN: FREQUENTLY ASKED QUESTIONS

1. **WHAT IS THE MOST IMPORTANT CONSIDERATION TO ENSURE PROGRESS?** Consistency in training is by far the most significant factor in the outcome.

2. **WILL A STRENGTH PROGRAM CAUSE ME TO GAIN WEIGHT?** The only way a human body can gain weight is to ingest more calories than it burns off. Lifting weights is an energy expenditure, so the act of lifting causes weight loss. Furthermore, post-exercise metabolism burn is higher when lifting is combined with more conditioning-type training methods than it is from endurance training alone. The key to not gaining weight for those struggling to maintain a weight class limit is to keep the eating appropriate and to keep the rep ranges conducive to power gains and not mass acquisition.

3. **CAN TRAINING WITH WEIGHTS MAKE ME SLOWER?** Absolutely, if your training is very slow, and your weight program is geared towards hypertrophy of slow twitch fibers. Training properly will enhance speed, which is why all sprinters on land, water, and ice do it.

4. **HOW OFTEN SHOULD I CHANGE THE PROGRAM?** The first weeks/months much of the gains made in strength are actually due to neurological efficiency, as opposed to gains in tissue strength. Therefore, novices can remain on a program a little longer than an advanced trainee. If a novice continues progressing after 4-6-8 weeks on a program, let them keep progressing. There would be no need to change the program. If they plateau, change the program. Trainees with more training years typically train hard for three weeks, followed by a lighter week.

5. **IF I AM SEVERELY TIME-RESTRICTED, WHAT ARE THE MOST BENEFICIAL EXERCISES I CAN DO TO MAXIMIZE BENEFIT?** First priority should be given to the areas of individual weakness that limit performance. For most, this would be speed. Resisted cord blitzes, retreats, lateral hops, and sprints all can be done in the dojo right after training. It doesn't get more efficient than that. In the gym, cleans (if done properly) are terrific. Squat variations provide a high return for the time it takes to do them. Variations of Split Squats and Split Squat Jumps may be the best of all.

6. **SHOULD I TRAIN BEFORE OR AFTER PRACTICE?** Train whenever you have to, to be most consistent. In an ideal world it would be done after practice, so the body has full energy for the training that most benefits performance (practice). Sessions can also be split up into morning and afternoon or evening sessions.

7. **IS THERE AN ORDER TO PROGRAMMING THE EXERCISES?** Every athlete should be warmed up and stretched out via mobility movements and/or stretching movements. Injury prevention exercises can contribute to that. After this initial phase all higher-velocity or heavier lifts like plyometrics, Olympic lifts, squats or deadlifts should be done. This is to ensure maximum freshness for the most taxing movements.

8. **MY BACK HURTS DOING CLEANS, SHOIULD I DO THEM ANYWAY?** Definitely not! The purpose of off-mat training is to improve performance. All of these exercises are merely tools. There are countless ways to change routines and combine exercises to make progress. We never want to create injuries off-mat. If cleans hurt, substitute dumbbell squat jumps in their place, and then go win the tournament anyway.

9. **HOW HEAVY SHOULD I LIFT?** The first set of every exercise should be a warm-up. After that, sets should be challenging but should never result in having missed a repetition. Even competitive lifters are wise to never miss reps. Karateka surely shouldn't be lifting so heavy that they fail.

10. **SHOULD I TEST MY STRENGTH LEVELS?** The big test is on the tournament mat. You should know by the training you do and the feedback of your coach and training partners if you're getting faster, and by the increase of weights lifted if you're getting stronger. Therefore, it is not imperative to test, and it's probably safer not to, but there is nothing wrong with periodic tests if you're prepared properly to do them.

11. **CAN I COMPETE SUCCESSFULLY WITHOUT STRENGTH TRAINING AND CONDITIONING?** Sure, not every great athlete in history was a hard-core overachiever outside of their sport practice. Some can get by without it and still perform admirably, although very few professional athletes do now. You just won't be your best.

3 Off-Mat Conditioning

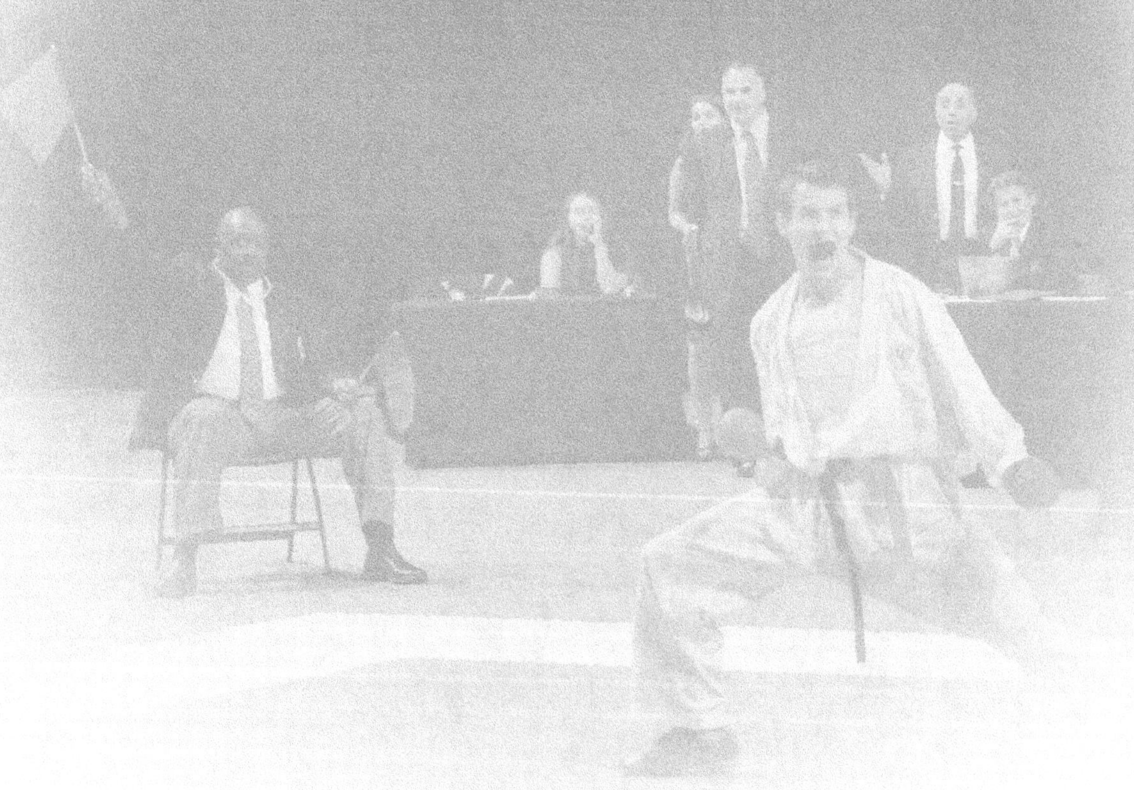

There are several components of functioning that can be enhanced by off-mat conditioning, including speed, speed-endurance and endurance.

Speed is typically prized by athletes and coaches of most all sports as the number one desired physical attribute. Without it, it is very hard to win, regardless of how biomechanically sound karate technique may be. It is therefore important to develop as much speed as possible. Much speed can be developed on-mat, but ideal speed optimization can occur only through a combination of on-mat and off-mat training. This is why all sprinters, cyclists, skaters, and swimmers who compete in sprint events seriously strength train.

In karate, speed is not enough. Because match scores at the highest levels are so close, matches are often won late. This match-winning score too often comes when one competitor is tired and thinking about being tired, and not fully engaged in tactics. Endurance is also essential to winning in karate. We must have both speed and speed-endurance to optimize our ability.

This need for the ability to repeatedly perform extremely high-intensity sport-specific movements is largely anaerobic, thus training for speed and speed-endurance would be greatly enhanced through high-intensity anaerobic training protocols. This is sport-specificity that was discussed previously. On-mat this might mean revolving partner drills in live kumite sparring, or simulated drills. Off-mat there are several options, including high-intensity interval training methods like running, circuiting exercises and/ or use of devices like stair climbers, stationary bikes, and rowing ergometers.

While aerobic contribution is typically not as high as anaerobic contribution in matches, and aerobic capacity is less important than anaerobic endurance, it should not be concluded that aerobic training is not beneficial, or worth any dedicated training time. The aerobic system cannot supply the incredible amount of energy required in a heated exchange in a match, but a strong aerobic base can enhance recovery from intermittent bouts of high-intensity exercise, both during a match, and between matches. This recovery is essential, because our competitor is free to initiate an attack at any time during a match, even after we have called off our attack because we were tired and unsuccessful. In summary, we need athletes that can strike fast like a rattlesnake and do so repeatedly. Thankfully, both speed and endurance can be developed in a very small amount of training time.

ESSENTIAL PRINCIPLES INHERRENT IN PROPER OFF-MAT CONDITIONING PROGRAMMING FOR KARATE ATHLETES

1. **MOST CONDITIONING SHOULD BE DONE ON-MAT IN A SPORT-SPECIFIC MANNER.** Proper conditioning training on-mat is the best way to increase endurance on-mat. If the training cycles are designed properly, the karateka should attain a high level of conditioning on-mat that is specific to the demands of the competition. This chapter will dive very deeply into this later on.

2. **SAFETY IS THE MOST IMPORTANT CONSIDERATION.** It goes without saying that athletes condition to get better at performance. Training for improved speed or endurance should never result in injuries that prevent an athlete from future training sessions. Warm-ups are critical and should include general total body warming, end range mobilization, activation

exercises, upcoming task-specifc movements and possibly some static stretches if desired. Reps of each drill should be allotted to warming up the ranges of motion required in the drills that are done at high speeds. Any drill that causes an athlete to function in poor mechanics should be omitted or avoided until safe mechanics can be maintained.

3. **OFF-MAT CONDITIONING MUST BE DONE IN AN EFFICIENT MANNER.** If there is an appropriate conditioning protocol on-mat during the training week, or several sessions, most karateka will not need a great deal of additional conditioning work off-mat, including high level competitors. Most would benefit greatly from as little as one session per week. That's a good thing because the first priority for enhancing perfprmance outcome is on-mat skill training. The second priority is conditioning for most. Priority three becomes power development through strength training. Doing all of this should leave very little time and energy left. One good conditioning session late in a week can be just the perfect amount to yield great benefits efficently. Because of fatigue, this one session should be as productive as possible in as little time as possible.

4. **USE A LOGICAL, SYSTEMATIC PROGRESSION.** Like all exercise formatting, all conditioning exercises should progress with each athlete fully safe, efficient and mechanically sound in each movement before introduction of a more complex skill. The risk of injury goes way down with slower progressions and an unyielding commitment to proper biomechanics. A good example is that an athlete should spend several weeks, or even months, training in a running program that progresses in intensity and speed, before runnning close to full speed.

5. **SPEED TRAINING SHOULD ONLY BE DONE WHEN THE BODY IS FRESH.** There is a huge difference between training for speed enhancement, and training for improved endurance. In fact, training for those qualities should be almost polar opposite programs. It is imposssible for a tired body to move at full speed. Always keep fresh in your mind that whenever you perform a motor skill, you are essentially "hitting save on that document." As we mentioned earlier, Physical Therapist Gray Cook says, "if your movement is poor, you're hitting save on a really bad document." Inversely, if you perform a terrific movement, you are "hitting save" on an exceptional pattern. A fatigued body rarely moves in optimal mechanics, and certainly cannot do so fast. To get fast, you have to be fast. Perform movements where you're trying to elicit a response of faster movement only when the body is rested. You simply cannot move fast when you're fatigued. Taking ample rest between reps is essential as well in training to become faster. Conversely, conditionning workouts should have very little rest and should be highly fatiguing.

6. **CONDITIONING IS BEST AFTER SKILL TRAINING AND LATE IN THE TRAINING WEEK.** A proper conditioning session should be quite exhausting. If a body is very exhausted, it can take days to recover. That means subsequent training sessions for several days can be impaired. A body cannot get faster if it is moving slower and improperly. Moving the hardest conditioning session to the end of the week, and just prior to the off day(s) affords the athlete the opportunity to have a high quality training week while improving on conditioning.

7. **SPEED AND ENDURANCE CAN BE IMPROVED IN THE SAME WORK-OUT.** This pursuit of enhancing speeed and endurance simultaneously may not be considered an optimal approach but may be appropriate for those with time constrictions, or those who cannot tolerate high volumes of training. That being said, if you one of these limiting circumstances and want to be faster and in better condition, a little trick for enhancing speed during a conditioning session is to use some speed development drills early on in a session (when the body is fresh) as a means to excite the nervous system. Examples can be low-level plyometrics, like jumping rope, speed/agility ladder drills, low box jumps and mini-hurdles. Once the speed work is completed succcessfully and the body starts to fatigue, conditioning work can start.

8. **SPEED DRILLS SHOULD BE FAIRLY SHORT IN DISTANCE AND DURATION.** Movement in karate is very intense, but not over a very long distance. The nature of practice and sparring renders a body to be near overtrained for many. The last thing a karateka needs is a pulled hamstring from running a full-speed 100 meter sprint, which is not specific to competition demands anyway. Karateka trying to improve their speed for blitzing would be much better served to run ten 10 meter runs at full speed, or 5 twenty meter runs, than they would to run one all out 100 meter sprint. This would obviously require significant rest intervals.

DESIGNING A PROGRAM

Much like the lifting program, we must assess time available for off-mat training and the needs of the individuals. For some, there may be a need for more speed. For others, time might be best spent on conditioning. Once we have assigned objectives, we need to assess how much time to allot to each.

It might be worth the time it takes to revisit the Bell Curve/Normal Distribution, when assessing performance needs:

FIGURE 52:

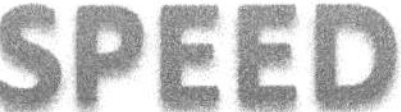

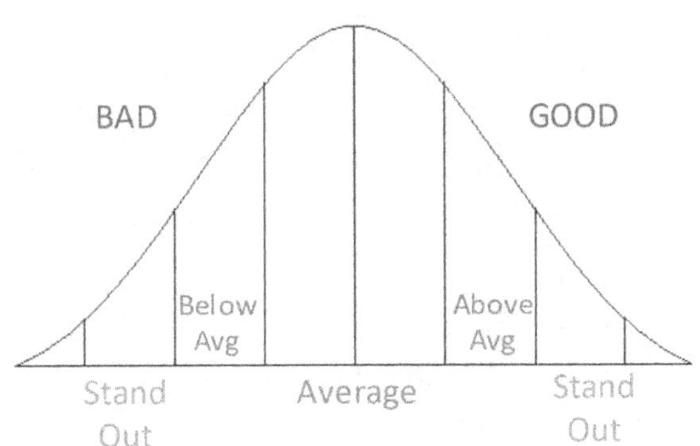

ENDURANCE/CONDITIONING

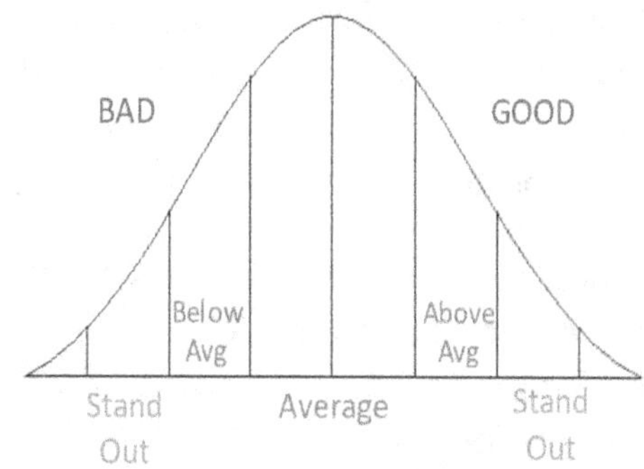

Where are you ?

PUTTING IT ALL TOGETHER

STEP 1

First, we need to assess the particular needs of the individual. Does the athlete need more speed when attacking, or retreating? Does the athlete need more conditioning? Is there concern about the ability to accelerate? Are backward and sideways movements where they should be in terms of both acceleration and speed? The list to assess here is long and should involve the karate coach, the athlete, and the strength and conditioning professional. The goal is to get a clear vision of what we are trying to achieve and what the end-product should look like. Only then can we design a map to get there.

STEP 2

Second, we have to determine the number of sessions per week the athlete can always make, without fail, and the amount of time needed per session. Remember, the number one factor contributing to success is the consistency and compliance in training. One session per week for a year will yield great gains in speed and endurance. Training too hard too fast and not sticking to a productive program because of fatigue or burn-out will not get desired results.

STEP 3

Once we determine both the amount of time per work-out and workouts per week, we can start designing the protocol. There are literally a countless number of exercises to choose from that can be combined into an infinite number of different protocols.

A sample template such as this one can now be designed. This would be for a competitor who will train off-mat once a week for an hour, in addition to the karate training sessions.

FIGURE 54:

PERIOD	TIME (Minutes)	OBJECTIVE
1	15	Warm-up, Mobility, Stretch
2	20	Fast Feet, Acceleration, Pure Speed
3	25	Conditioning

In this hypothetical model, our athlete will spend one hour, once a week, on a track in supplemental conditioning. This session leaves ample warm up time, time for speed development and finishes with a strong conditioning component. This is a very efficient means of training.

A sample of a daily program may therefore look like this:

FIGURE 55:

<u>FRIDAY</u> - on track
1. Foam roll: 1 minute each:
    a.   quads
    b.   IT bands
    c.   groins
    d.   glutes
    e.   hamstrings
    f.   calves
2. Mobilities: 1x 15 meters each
    a.   Knee to Chest Walk
    b.   Leg Cradles
    c.   Backwards hamstring (slowly)
    d.   Quads
    e.   Lateral Groin – both directions
    f.   Quad with RDL
    g.   Cross Over Toe Touch – both directions
2. Foam Roll: same as above, 30 seconds each
3. Stretch: as needed
4. Speed running drills: 2x5 meters each, maximizing number of reps per 5 meters and speed of reps
    a.   fast feet forward
    b.   fast feet sideways
    c.   low high knees, toes in
    d.   low high knees, toes out
    e.   ankling
    f.   high knees
    g.   butt kicks
    h.   A-skip (knee punch emphasis)
    i.   A-skip (ground strike emphasis)
    j.   Skip for height
    k.   B-skip
    l.   high knee carioca
    m.   tuck jump into sprint
6. Sled Sprints: 5x15 meters at full speed, with 1 minute rest between reps
7. 6x200 meters, 4-5 seconds off projected best time, 2 minutes rest between reps.
8. Roll and stretch well

FINAL THOUGHTS: FREQUENTLY ASKED QUESTIONS

1. **WHAT ARE POTENTIAL PITFALLS TO ADDING A RUNNING WORKOUT TO THE TRAINING WEEK?** Getting injured is always a concern for karate athletes because the nature of their training in a combat sport already exposes them to significantly higher incidence of injury. There are some potential concerns and safety measures that should be implemented in the best interest of the athletes. First, have very high standards for the quality of movement in the warmups. Warmups must be both intentional and thorough. The last thing an athlete needs is a pulled hamstring that causes missed time on the mat. Second, make sure not to sprint all out on sprints until the body has had a significant amount of training time to prepare for such high intensity bursts. This will help reduce chance of muscle pulls as well. Third, give more rest than you are inclined to give during speed development drills so the nervous system and muscle can work safely and at speeds needed to promote increased speed. Do not blend speed development work into conditioning blocks of the session. Fourth, don't overtrain during the conditioning sessions.

2. **IS THERE A MEANS TO REGULATE THE VOLUME OF ENDURANCE WORK OUTS AND AVOID OVERTRAINING?** Yes, counting the total distance of intervals is one simple measure. A good starting point might be 800-900 meters, which can be broken down many ways, such as:

   a. 3x300
   b. 4x200
   c. 6x150
   d. 9x100
   e. 2x200-2x150-2x100
   f. 3x200-3x100.

   Once the athlete's body has settled into this volume (typically in 3 weeks) more distance can be added.

3. **WOULDN'T INTERVAL TRAINING 3 TIMES A WEEK INCREASE FITNESS OVER A ONCE-A-WEEK PROGRAM?** Yes, track runners typically do interval runs or tempo runs, depending on the event(s) more than once a week, but they don't do so in a beat-up physical state, caused by intense karate practice. Remember, our goal is not to be in track runner shape, it's to be in better karate shape than our competitors or our current self.

4. **SHOULD I RUN BEFORE OR AFTER PRACTICE?** Typically, one should condition at the end of the week, after practice so the body is not fatigued for the most important training sessions, the on-mat ones. In extreme cases needing much speed development, a low volume, high quality session could precede the on-mat training week, just after a day off, so that the body is fully fresh.

5. **CAN I COMPETE SUCCESSFULLY WITHOUT OFF-MAT CONDITIONING?** Sure, not every great athlete in history was a hard-core overachiever outside of their sport practice. Some can get by without it and still perform admirably, although very few professional athletes do now. You just won't be your best.

On-Mat Conditioning

4

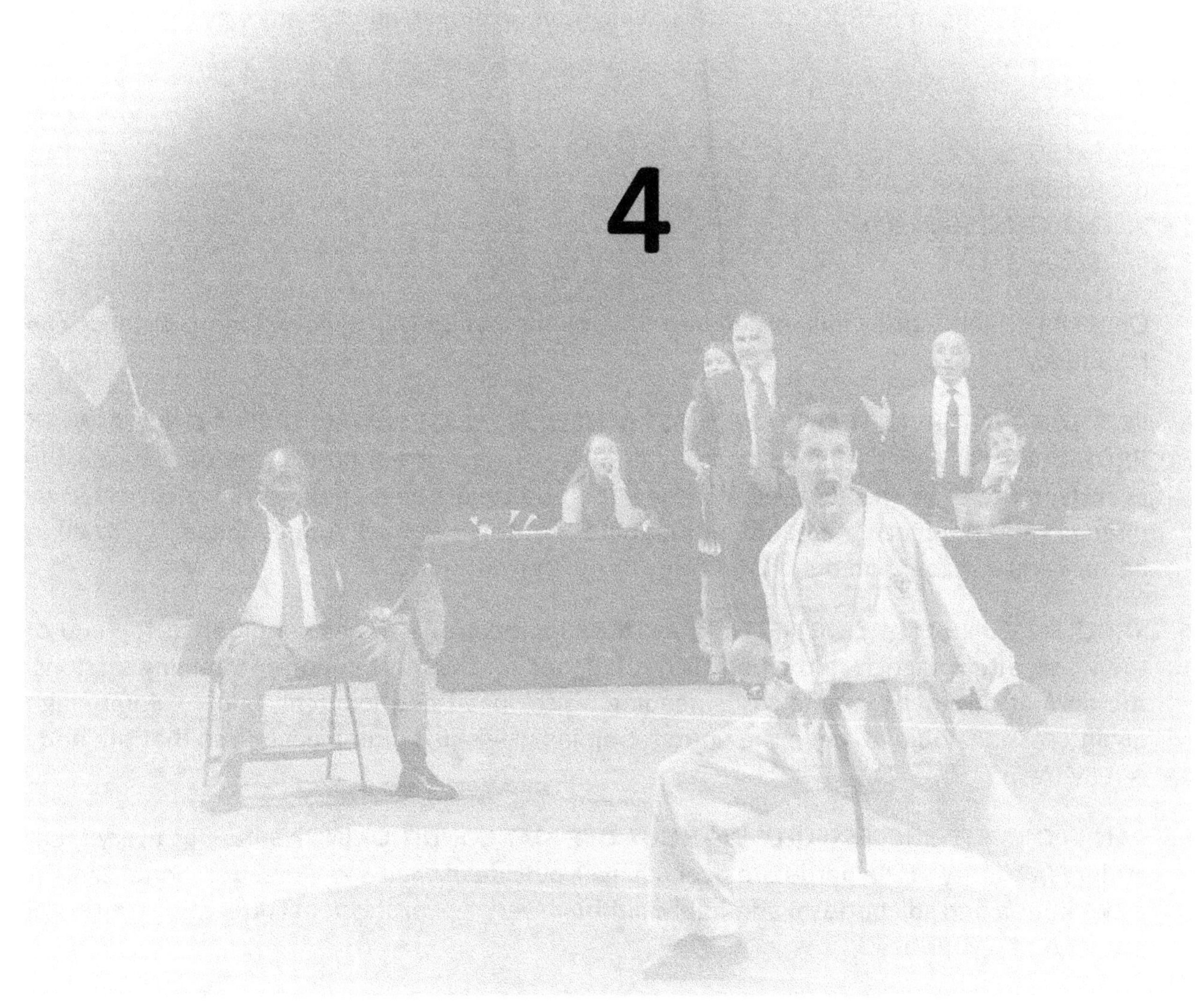

INTRODUCTION

Note: this is a critically important contributor to overall karate performance, perhaps the most significant contributor. Without adequate strength, speed, and endurance even the karateka with perfect technique cannot win, and neither can the one that can run 100-mile endurance races if their body is trained merely to tolerate a long, slow, oxidative test. Therefore, this chapter will be a deep dive into on-mat conditioning.

Of all traits that contribute to performance, not including the techniques of kicking, punching, and timing of strikes, conditioning is typically agreed upon by most coaches and athletes as the most important contributor to performance outcome. It is likely that everyone knowledgeable in the sport would say it is critical to have great conditioning.

One method to attain the great physiological benefits of increased endurance, aerobic power, capillary density, mitochondrial density, enzymatic benefits, enhanced metabolic energy stores and favorable body composition changes is to do so through purely aerobic activity. Examples would be jogging or using aerobic-based machines such as stair climbers and bicycles. While this can provide some of the aforementioned benefits, it is probably not the most conducive method of providing significant performance changes in karate matches. The body adapts to the training stimulus, hence "the body becomes its function." Slow aerobic work is far from the specificity of karate performance. We certainly don't want slow, methodical fighters with no ability to burst.

A better approach in terms of enhancing conditioning for karate might be to do tempo or interval training. Karate is largely an anaerobic sport, consisting of many ultra-high-intensity and explosive bursts. Depending on the exercise prescription, bodily adaptations from a properly constructed anaerobic training program can include increases in speed, power, change of direction, agility, economy of movement, neuromuscular, musculoskeletal, cardiovascular, and endocrine functions, bone density, connective tissue strength and metabolic capacity among other benefits. This would seem to provide more to the end performance than merely jogging several miles. This is the reason why many track coaches prescribe a protocol including tempo training, such as four reps of 4-minute runs, or a high intensity interval training program such as a forty-five-second-high intensity movement, followed by 45-135 second rest interval. An off-mat program of running intervals thus would be very beneficial, but is it the most beneficial way to condition a karate athlete?

Many exercise physiologists and strength and conditioning coaches might successfully argue that although physiological changes will certainly be gained from running intervals, there is a better way, one which is more specific to tournament performance, and more specific to karate performance; on-mat, high intensity interval training., appropriately using karate techniques in a well-designed circuit.

SKILL TRAINING IS NOT CONDITIONING, CONDITIONING IS CONDITIONING

It is important to distinguish the difference between technique improvement (skill acquisition), speed acquisition training and conditioning. Both skill and speed acquisition modalities should consist of very short, perfectly executed (skill acquisition) near full speed (speed acquisition) work intervals, with very long rest intervals. The work to rest ratio may be 1:12 or as high as 1:20. The reason is because the body cannot move most efficiently or quickly if it is tired. If the body is tired it will move slower. You cannot get faster by moving slower. Likewise, if the body is tired, it will often resort to compromised mechanics. You cannot attain great technique by repeatedly engraining bad technique. Therefore, speed acquisition and skill acquisition drills should both be of the highest quality, with long rest intervals to ensure freshness. Conversely, the body has to become tired to enhance fitness, so work to rest ratios in drills designed to improve conditioning can be very exhaustive, such as a work to rest ratio of 1:1, like running hard for thirty seconds and resting for thirty to sixty seconds. This means that the speed or skill acquisition methods would essentially be a polar opposite approach to the conditioning approach.

While on-mat training may be hard at times, it won't likely optimize conditioning unless it is built into a specific protocol. Conditioning is hard, so intense that it probably should not be done more than once or twice a week for more than 20-40 minutes. Heart rates will get high, minds will fatigue, lactate and hydrogen will flood the muscles and cause significant burning in the muscles. It's not easy to recover from it. For those reasons, an athlete should do these intense on-mat drills at the end of practice and never before, especially not before skill acquisition, timing, or speed drills. The body will not get faster when it is severely fatigued and catabolic. Sensei's can yell all they want; it still will result in a tired muscle not capable of moving faster or enhancing speed. Therefore, in establishing a fully comprehensive training program, one might consider doing speed-enhancement and skill acquisition early in the practice when the body is fresh and conditioning late in the practice, and at the end of the week.

A SUPERIOR METHOD OF ON-MAT CONDITIONING

There are numerous benefits of anaerobic training, and they are superior to long slow distance training for karate performance. We've seen that running provides many benefits, although it lacks specificity. Sparring is often used as a conditioning method and is very beneficial. It is taxing, sport-specific and makes an athlete focus during times of duress. This is critical for the athlete and must be done. It is not however, the only way to condition and should probably not be the only method of on-mat conditioning. The fact is that way too many athletes get hurt during all-out dojo wars that we all love so much. An injured athlete is not one that is bettering their performance. There is another way to derive the benefits of aerobic exercise, and interval training that is sport-specific, and most importantly, keeps the risk of injury lower: the creation of circuits that include sport-specific movements mixed with resisted movements and/or running or bodyweight exercises that elicit strength responses or significantly higher heart rates.

An example might be:

CIRCUIT: 30 seconds each station, rest 3 minutes after each round, 2-4 times through the circuit
   a. Kettlebell goblet alternating leg lunges.
   b. Heavy bag continuous striking
   c. Plank Hold
   d. Resisted Cord Blitzing
   e. Defending strikes while trapped in a corner.
   f. Vision Training Drill
   g. Lateral Movement footwork drill

The number of contributing exercises one can choose from is immense, the combinations of circuits one can construct is infinite.

PHILOSOPHY FOR ALL IN DESIGNING AN ON-MAT TRAINING PROGRAM

If you have read this far, you have read scientifically sound information on conditioning and training. Now the subject is what you should do on the mat. That depends upon your physiology: your strengths, weaknesses, and areas which you can concentrate on to yield the highest change in performance over the least amount of time.

The first thing you have to do, is determine what equipment you have access to in the dojo, what equipment you need that you can purchase, and what fits within the confines of your training philosophy, space allotment, current activity level of training, past training history, likes, dislikes, needs and time available. You obviously should not create a program that includes heavy lifting exercises if you're already lifting on other days. Likewise, you shouldn't program extensive amounts of medicine ball throws if they are typically done in karate training workouts.

Once this is done, the physiology needs to be assessed. A slow or weak fighter (one who struggles to initiate a more explosive attack or retreat) will need to prioritize movements that increase explosiveness, thus they may include things like dumbbell squat jumps, dumbbell step up jumps, split squat jumps, plyometric box hops, etc., if the dojo has these dumbbells to use. These are "core" components to the design of the circuit. Conversely, an explosive fighter that tires more easily may skip these exercises and concentrate more on conditioning movements, like stations of more karate specific movements, like doing all out attacks to a heavy bag (with proper technique) in a manner where rest is low, and effort is high. There's much more to this than just making everyone do the same thing because you have drills that "make them tired". If tired was a worthy goal, the athlete could carry the 1,100-pound strongman yoke 30 yards for time. That athlete would indeed be tired, but it would have nothing to do with karate.

Once the items you have available to use, and the needs are assessed, allot a percentage of time to very specific movements versus the non-specific things you will do. For example, for the weak, or slower fighter, we previously mentioned resisted jumping. Maybe you are doing a circuit of 8 exercise for thirty seconds. Plug those in first. Then plug in more specific karate exercises.

As for prescribing long lists of specific drills, this area is too subject to change. What is needed by one competitor is not needed by another, thus the ability to self-evaluate and self-prescribe is a preferred method. For example, do you remember the scorpion kick craze? Everyone got on the band wagon to train this drill. But is that skill for everyone? No. For highly specific karate drills you may consider incorporating, you may wish to look at George Kotaka's Web site Kumite Academy at www.kumiteacademy.com. He provides a wonderful approach to drills moving from fundamentals to advanced training.

The circuit design may therefore start out as:

CIRCUIT: 3x through, 30 seconds per station, no rest between sets, rest 2 minutes per round
1. Dumbbell squat jumps
2. Resisted cord blitz
3. DB Split Squat Jumps
4. Resisted Cord Retreat into Attack

Once the more specific exercises are added, it may morph to look like this:

CIRCUIT: 3x through, 30 seconds per station, no rest between sets, rest 2 minutes per round
1. Dumbbell squat jumps
2. Heavy bag gyaku-zuki as many as possible
3. Resisted cord blitz
4. Alternating leg mawashi-geri Jodan
5. DB Split Squat Jumps
6. Shadow sparring with partner facing you but remaining 10 feet away from each other
7. Resisted Cord Retreat into Attack
8. Trapped in corner defending continual attacks from a partner.

This will provide the conditioning effect specific to the demands of tournament matches (4 minutes of high intensity). If done hard, it will be more strenuous than a match, because there is no "re-set" time where attacks are broken off to re-group. In this model there are many movements to enhance explosion, and half of the circuit are direct karate techniques. Note, some athletes may need more karate techniques and others more physiology-changing movements.

DISTINGUISHING BETWEEN THE NOVICES/INTERMEDIATES AND THE ELITES

The goal of program design is to closely match the program design with the needs of the individuals. This can be better accomplished if it is also specific to the level of the trainee. While we cannot prescribe an individualized program for everyone, especially without assessing them, we can plant the seed of designing on-mat conditioning programs from a philosophical basis by breaking them down simply into generic groups.

BEGINNERS:
1. Program should be easy.
2. Program should promote enhanced fitness, but also be fun and something valued as helpful.
3. Trainee must be consistent to approve.
4. Simple, non-complicated movements should be prescribed. For example, kettlebell goblet squats would be a preferred choice over squats, dumbbell split squat jumps, power cleans, squats and other more complex movements.
5. Proper technique is essential.
6. No risks should be taken.
7. Bodyweight or light weights should be used.
8. Plan with the mindset that anything will benefit the novice.

INTERMEDIATES:
1. Program should still be fun.
2. Consistency is still the highest priority.
3. Trainees should be able to provide feedback on exercises they feel they need.
4. Proper technique is still essential.
5. Trainees can increase weights to very challenging ones.
6. Complexity of movements can be increased.
7. Some individualization can occur.

ELITES:

This is an entirely different animal. This has to be very precise, as the difference between competitors at the international level is miniscule. It's hard to be this precise, and there is so much more to consider. What follows here is a deep dive, like real deep! It may seem overly deep, and is definitely so for most, but not for the fighter with international skills that overachieves, has serious goals that are hard to reach, and is willing to pay the price to make them come true. Let's start that deep dive.

Maybe you can start by ask yourself the question "what do the very best karate competitors have in common. How do people who have won multiple world championship approach their preparation and competition?

What do all-time greats like Rafael Aghayev, Alexandre Biamonte, Stefano Maniscalco, and Wayne Otto have in common, or on the women's side Roberta Dominici, Ayumi Uekusa, Mariam Elezaby, Kate Sung, and Laurence Fischer? How about current greats like Steven Da Costa, Irina Zaretska and Milo Miyahara? And what did all-time greats here in the USA, like George Kotaka, Tom Scott, Elissa Au, and Shannon Nishi do? Surely there are few areas in common. What skills have they displayed? How have they achieved those skills? Ask yourself, "where am I in relationship to them?"

FIGURE 56:

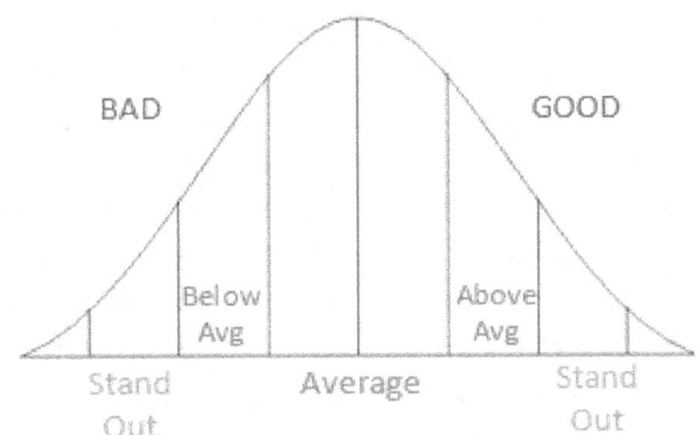

Now onto the promised deep dive considerations in designing elite programs:

CONSIDERATION #1: KNOW THYSELF, EVALUATE THYSELF, GET EVALUATED

One of the most important attributes for every elite athlete is the ability to see themselves and their strengths and weaknesses. Socrates said, "to know thyself is the beginning of wisdom." Socrates, humbly insisted that "if he was wise, it was only because he recognized his own ignorance." This is one of the most important areas to work on, to see yourself objectively, understanding what you do well, and what you need to work on.

Once you know who you are, it is easier to pick drills for both skill acquisition and in creating a sport-specific circuit. There are several different types of fighters, and they can all win with drastically different styles. Can you identify your style as one of these three styles? (This is from Antonio Oliva Seba, seminars.) Sensei Oliva is recognized as "one of the pioneers of martial arts and world leader in tactics for combat sports." If you can recognize your style. You can then devise training needs to enhance your style.

For example, an "aggressive fighter", especially one that fights "strong," might want to use sprint drills and more work on the legs for speed. This might mean more pure speed drills in earlier stages of practice and resisted cord or squat jump resisted movements during the conditioning circuit, where they can move at somewhat higher velocities. Why? Because he is strengthening his weaknesses or eliminating them.

The "Intellectual fighter" might want to work on timing and reaction drills as some of the stations in the circuit. They are different types of fighters, with different strengths and weaknesses, and should train differently. Assessing your fighting style into one of Oliva's three groups can help you to better determine more of your needs.

1. **Tendencies of the "Emotional, Aggressive or Attacker"**
   Attacking fighters keep attacking, and if they are not successful, they attack harder and harder, thus they burn a lot of energy and can benefit from strength-endurance drills to aid in economy of movement. If they do not succeed when attacking, they feel like a failure. They are typically very aggressive, good at attacks, but often times weaker on defense, especially when moving backwards and to the side. Movement drills would be good for them in the circuit. Some have also said these athletes have a "strong body but no brain," or, "they have a brain but do not use it as they should". This might indicate the need for drills on explosive movement, drills on attacking at angles that work on footwork specific to that and drills on recovery, with that foot work as well. Since they are strong, they can reduce heavy strength training protocols, as the emphasis on movement will yield a greater gain in overall performance ability. Speed drills would be very valuable, since their style i sone of attacking.

2. **Tendencies of the "Intellectual Fighter"**
   These fighters are typically calculating. They are more likely to counter fight, are typically not as strong, but they are very clever. They are usually great at defense and difficult to score on. They usually possess good coordination but do not fight strong. Although they often are very clever, they are not as focused on winning as much as "not losing. The approach for exercise

prescription here should be drills on vision, with an emphasis on explosive leg capabilities. Recommended exercises would include resisted cord use for lateral movements and blitzing, perhaps with a reactive component, such as a technique or two thrown by a training partner serving as uke. Squat jumps, step up jumps, split squat jumps and lateral hops would be dynamic movements that can help increase functional power.

3. **Tendencies of the "Dynamic fighter", or "Methodical fighter".**
   These athletes can do both the attacking and intellectual styles. This karateka is very athletic, with a good body and brain, and is very balanced between attacking and defending., They are typically emotionally cool, and use both aggressive fighter and intellectual fighter drills. Their approach is more of a hybrid style on-mat and off-mat.

   Continuing on in getting to know thyself, the following questions may be some very high-level, sport-specific thought-provokers, unique to elite level karate, for your self-evaluation, and the evaluation from your coach/sensei. These can be very beneficial and provide a competitive advantage over other who do not self-assess on a level this deep.

   1. Is your focus continually on the present, and can you remain there without getting distracted by the future or past? If you struggle here, incorporate some drills into your off days, or during rest intervals in your conditioning circuits that can improve this. It might sound a bit extreme, but if you did a few minutes of concentrated work on improving focus during times you'd be resting anyway, at the end of a year you'd have accumulated many hours of time spent strengthening a weakness. It may no longer be a weakness. The gains of a few minutes of daily work may be nominal, but the summation of nominal gains can be substantial.

   2. Is your ability to move, in all directions, to get you in and out of trouble as good as your competitors? If not, drills to help this can be part of early skill acquisition in practice, and if done well technically, they can be done within conditioning sessions. If this is your strength, you may reduce use of them in conditioning sessions in order to put more effort into other exercises that will yield more gains.

   3. Are you sound in your match preparation to score? Unless you are the fastest competitor, you will need to "set-up the score" in matches. Drills to help this can become part of your circuit. One example is to create new ways through timing or movement in resisted cords to set up your favorite attack.

   4. Is your explosion, in all directions, better than your opponents? If not, you would benefit from more exercises to develop that trait. If this is a deficiency you can include more plyometrics or functional resisted movements in your conditioning protocol. Many times programs designed to enhance explosion are done only jumping upwards and never laterally or horizontally.

5. Is your execution of technique biomechanically sound? If it is, great. If not, and your physical attributes are solid, you may decrease strength and conditioning a bit and spend more time on mechanics.

6. Do you recover well when scoring or breaking off an attack? You'll need speed both going forward and backwards and can tailor the program to improve in those areas.

You can now see why it is of paramount importance to know thyself.

This knowledge becomes critically important when designing the sport-specific program. As mentioned, the big, strong dojo bully likely doesn't need a great amount of heavy strength training. There is no one magical program that optimizes performance for all fighters. For example, a fighter working an insane number of hours to improve his bench press from 300 pounds to 315 pounds isn't going to display a difference in a kumite match, or kata for that matter. Conversely, the weak fighter than exhibits great stamina but isn't explosive enough would seem to benefit more from gaining explosive power in the weightroom. It is therefore essential to know thyself as a fighter, and as a physiological being. This way the circuit can be tailored for each type of fighter. The aggressive fighter can include less lifting, and more defensive and reactionary skills (in a conditioning protocol, not for speed enhancement or skill acquisition.) Likewise, the conditioning circuit of the intellectual fighter can de-emphasize the defensive reaction drills in the circuit and increase the strength and power components.

CONSIDERATION #2: THE PHYSIOLOGICAL TRAIT OF VISION

Distance is vital in kumite. Most of the time when a technique is thrown too far away, there is no score. Too often when the technique thrown is too close, the result is a penalty.

This is true in all sports. In football the quarterback drops back and lofts a pass that falls perfectly into the receiver's arms. If the pass is too long or too short, the result is an incompletion, or possibly even an interception. This scene is more about vision and dept perception than arm strength.

You can imagine, or rather you should imagine, as many sports as you can that rely on vision and depth perception.

Here is an excerpt from an interview with David Epstein, author of *The Sports Gene*.

Epstein states, "It turns out that even the best baseball hitters in the world have perfectly pedestrian reaction times." Doesn't that blow your mind? We all assume their reaction times would be many times better than the rest of us, but they don't. Interestingly, author David Epstein actually scored better on a visual reaction time test than Albert Pujols did. If you're not a serious baseball fan, Albert was an 11x All-Star, 3x Most Valuable Player, 2x World Series Champion, 6x Silver Slugger Award Winner, 2x Gold Glove winner, and those are only about half of his accolades.

"It turns out that even the best baseball hitters in the world have perfectly pedestrian reaction times."

If it's not their reflexes, what is it?

The Los Angeles Dodgers tested the vision of their players to see if vision itself was a factor. They found that the average professional baseball player has a tested vision of 20/15. Half of their team was at 20/10, meaning that they can see perfectly clear at 20 feet what normal people can only see clearly at ten feet. Some players were 20/9 and one was 20/8.

According to Epstein, baseball batters pick up on cues from the pitcher's body before their release of the pitch. Without pitchers knowing it, the hitters are actually focusing in on the motion of the pitcher's shoulder and the pitcher's torso and hand, and then as soon as the ball's released on what's called the flicker (which is a flashing pattern that the red seams make as they rotate), the hitters were picking up those anticipatory cues that allows them to hit the ball. Surprisingly, the reaction time of major league hitters was not the cause of success and was theorized. Believe it or not, teachers, lawyers and doctors all displayed the same approximate visual stimulus (about 200 milliseconds). That's one-fifth of a second.

That's half the total transit time of a fastball. We simply do not have a biological system that is capable of tracking objects moving at that speed. So once the ball is halfway to the hitter, he might as well close his eyes. He's already swinging wherever he's swinging. In that first half of the pitch, right when the ball's out of the hand, the hitter has to have picked up cues from the pitcher's body and the movement of the ball to know where it's going ahead of time. It is not that professional athletes are reacting more quickly, it's that they're reading the picture they're seeing and anticipating where the ball is going to be. It's like it's the software, not the hardware, right? They can do that because they are genetically gifted visually.

This need for superior vision is true in nearly all sports; it requires vision and attention to see what is coming at you. Muhammed Ali, considered by many as "the greatest of all time", said, "Float like a butterfly, sting like a bee." We've all heard that for decades, but do you know what came after that line? It was this line, "The hands can't hit what the eyes don't see."

So, what is required for the vision of the karate fighter? Can a fighter improve their vision and change their performance? The answer is unequivocally, yes.

What Is Sports Vision Training?

Athletes are always looking for an extra edge to help them perform better at their sport. You've probably thought about aerobic capacity, endurance, strength, muscle tone and flexibility. But karate is a sport where split-second timing can make all the difference, and exceptional visual skills are a must. Science has shown in many studies that professional athletes have much better depth perception, hand-eye coordination, and other visual skills than non-athletes.

Sports vision can definitely be improved, just like strength, speed, or endurance. Sports vision training can take the good to exceptional, with a program that actually trains your vision to a point where you can truly excel in your sport. Talent, training, and commitment get you far.

Is this really effective, or all theoretical?

Eric Schlopy was a three-time Olympic skier, who had won a bronze medal in the world championships, two medals in the World Cup and seven National championships. In a personal conversation, he revealed that he had a horrific fall in an international championship race in Japan, and it nearly destroyed his career. He was unable to compete for several years while he was healing. He said that the only thing he could work on was visual training and visualization, from which he concluded vision training was more valuable to his competition than lessons in mechanics. That is powerful information. Think about that. A skier who improved his skiing without skiing. It's a testament to his desire, fortitude, and intelligence to find a way to win under extreme adversity and to persevere through this seemingly impossible challenge.

Reflexion.com is a premier authority on sports vision training. Their research has shown that it is possible to improve in many aspects of sight. This comes from their organization:

"A sports visual exercise or therapy will focus on some or all of the individual vision skills needed for them to reach their highest playing abilities.

- Eye Tracking: learning to keep your eye on the object
- Peripheral Awareness: the ability to see things out of the corner of your eye
- Dynamic Visual Acuity: learning to see objects clearly while they're in motion
- Focusing: changing focus from one object to another quickly and clearly
- Hand-eye and Body-eye Coordination: being able to use your eyes to direct the movements of hands, body, and other specific limbs.
- Depth Perception: quickly and accurately judging the distance and speed of something
- Reaction Time: the rate at which you can perceive a visual event and react to stimulus
- Contrast Sensitivity: the ability to distinguish between an object and the background
- Balance: ability to stay upright and in control of body movement

As you can see, there are a lot of visual skills that apply to many different sports – and they are all essential and affect each one differently. Learning your strengths and weaknesses in each of these areas can prove to make a massive difference in how you train."

Remember, not seeing things can cause a serious consequence in this sport!

The International Sports Vision Association has detailed needs for vision skills specific to boxing, which would certainly benefit karate fighters:

Anticipation Timing

Since timing is the key to effective performance, knowing the right time to throw a punch is very crucial. It is also important not to over-commit yourself in response to an opponent's feints.

Concentration

It is essential to be able to focus through distraction and maintain a high level of concentration throughout the bout, not allowing crowd noise, flashing lights or an opponent's taunting to be a distraction from the task at hand. A slight deficiency or lapse in concentration can mean mental or physical error, which could mean the loss of a bout- or worse- injury.

Depth Perception

The ability to deliver an effective blow is much more complicated than it may appear to the casual observer. It involves a snapping and twisting motion that makes it necessary to determine the exact distance of an opponent in order to deliver the blow with maximum power.

Eye-Hand/Body/Foot Coordination

Total coordination is essential to the maintenance of good balance. Fighters, therefore, have an obvious need to integrate a sense of balance with the visual motor system. Eye-Hand coordination is also one of the keys to landing effective punches within the scoring range.

Eye Fatigue

Boxing is a very fatiguing sport, especially when both fighters are evenly matched in weight, skills, and conditioning. Professional bouts for championships can go 15 three-minute rounds. With only a one-minute rest between rounds, physical fatigue is guaranteed. This drain of energy can greatly affect concentration, visual reaction time and eye-hand coordination. Eye fatigue can also affect performance levels in much the same way. When the muscles in our eyes feel tired or strained, we feel the fatigue all over. Just as we use weightlifting routines to improve physical endurance levels, we can also use a program of visual exercises to enhance your eye muscles, and thereby reduce fatigue."

Visual Assessment

Your visual system definitely affects how you score that perfect gyaku-zuki; you have to be on the proper line of attack the Sei Chu Sen, and that requires visual acuity and depth perception.

To gain a greater understanding of your visual system, you should certainly get an assessment from a sports vision doctor. They will seek answers to several questions, such as are you left or right-eye dominant? What is your vision? How well do your eyes work as a team? Are you right or left-handed? These questions and many more, along with testing, will reveal important aspects of your visual system and what you can do to improve your visual skills. Back to the idea of knowing yourself.

Once you have an understanding of your own visual system, you can use prescribed training exercises to benefit your performance. This may even change some of your tactical methods. For example, if you are right-eye dominant, you might do a variety of attacks and counters differently than if you are left-eye dominant.

Vision Training for the Karateka

A great time to include vision training exercises would be during the rest intervals of the circuit. Remember, we may be doing a 4-minute sport-specific tempo circuit on a 1:1 work to rest ratio. Instead of checking out mentally and physically during the rest interval, a karateka can enhance visual skills during the rest intervals. Likewise, these vision drills can be used in the circuit itself to lower a heartrate that is excessively high. Like focus training, merely adding minutes daily into the rest interval times can a huge benefit in match performance via the summation of nominal gains.

Improvements can be seen in speed and accuracy of eye movements, dynamic visual acuity, hand-eye coordination, eye tracking and focusing, peripheral vision, fusion flexibility, and stamina [the ability to keep both eyes working together under high speed or physically stressful situations], depth perception, reaction time and visualization. This results in a finely tuned visual system, which helps you learn to anticipate and respond more quickly to complex situations.

While some may explore the option to get professional guidance, others may opt to try and create a DIY beneficial protocol on their own. Here are a few traits you can enhance.

Depth Perception

This visual ability enables you to make spatial judgments, including how far away an object or person is from you, and the velocity it may be traveling towards you That obviously is critical for fighters being attacked, especially when you're an intellectual fighter, fighting an attacking opponent. Some of this ability depends strictly on physical characteristics. For example, spacing between the center of your two pupils (pupillary distance) is thought to play a major role in how well you see in three dimensions. Regardless of your genetic gifts, this is essential for a fighter to excel at. Vision (sport vision), in kumite is vital, you must be able to intuitively know if you are in range or out of range. Rafael Aghayev was a master at this. Think of him bouncing calmly in the corner, just where we would all want our opponents most of the time. But he was comfortable there and had great depth perception on the distance of his opponents, and how fast they were moving. This provided him with the correct timing to attack or counter-attack.

One simple way to train for this skill is to research on the computer eye training exercises that promote identifying objects or shapes that are in random, dot-patterned backgrounds. The website SAS Blogs has sensational puzzles for this. Another simple quick tip that can be done in the dojo involves a simple pen drill. Have you ever tried to put the cap on a pen and miss? Practicing this skill at arm's length is one way to improve your depth perception. Do it with both eyes open, each eye closed, standing on two legs, then one, or rotating your head laterally while doing it. Another method is to hold a very small pebble or BB at arm's length and drop it into a drinking straw, or practice threading a needle. All of these, and others you can research or create can be done during the conditioning circuit, or between rounds. These drills are far superior to sitting around, texting, between rounds.

Another idea might be to hang a balloon or small ball from the ceiling using rope. Hang the ball so that is hangs approximately 2 feet from the ceiling. Use your hands to bat the balloon or beach ball back and forth from left to right. This will help your eyes focus on precisely where an object is.

Or perhaps you could use a flashlight in a dark room. Take a flashlight and have a family member or friend make patterns on the wall. Patterns should go to the left, right, up, down, and diagonally. Follow the patterns closely with your eyes. If you're fortunate, you can find a good karate-specific professional and try using a light system like Fitlight. For example, at the Champion

Sports Performance at the Southfork Sports Complex, Coach Chris Stratis has served USA Karate and their elite athletes for years. He has had great success in helping karate athletes improve their sports vision using Fitlight. These are great devices and available on the internet.

Hand and Eye Dominance.

Understanding which eye dominates may also help an athlete adopt better strategies for improving athletic performance.

Most karate athletes know they are either right-handed or left-handed, and they try to quickly learn how to compete from both sides. But they may not realize that their dominant eye may process visual information more fully and accurately than their non-dominant eye. For instance, the question can be asked: if you are right-handed but left eye dominant, what does that do to your ability to fight left-handed? You have spent your life building a library of neurons that convey distance based on the dominant eye and its position. Knowing which eye dominates can help an athlete achieve better head and eye positioning to interpret fast action in Kumite.

Handedness and eye-dominance are undoubtedly associated statistically, although a previous meta-analysis has found that the precise relationship is difficult to explain, with about 35% of right-handers and 57% of left-handers being left eye dominant.

Some athletes are cross-dominant, meaning that a right-handed person is left-eye dominant, or a left-handed person is right-eye dominant. This can be an advantage in some sports, but potentially a serious disadvantage in sports such as archery and target shooting where one side of the body is used to both aim and shoot. Kumite has similarities to shooting, so studying that might benefit the most serious of competitors.

In kumite, a dominant hand and dominant eye tend to work together much more efficiently when they are on the same side of the body. So, if you have trouble perceiving the distance with your technique, cross dominance might be the reason. This can be evident if you are not receiving points because you are too far away of if you receive a lot of penalties for contact, (but that was not your intent).

You may need to make adjustments, such as switching your stance. You can still fight from a left hand or right-hand stance but you will need to turn your chest a little so your dominant eye can provide the necessary distance to you.

It sounds a little crazy, but some studies have shown that balance training helps peripheral vision and improves our ability to recognize movement cues quicker. Perhaps your rest intervals can incorporate a balancing activity during the vision training? Vision is an appropriate segue to move to ways to enhance your timing.

CONSIDERATION #3: THE PHYSIOLOGICAL TRAIT OF TIMING

Timing is the ability to coincide movements in relation to external factors. Timing is a combination of vision, as we mentioned earlier with the professional baseball players, decision-making, coordination, and reaction time. If you want to split the timing of an attack you must be able to perceive the distance and time the movement, so you strike exactly as they get in range.

One of the best ways to improve timing is to see a lot of drills and participate in kumite. Referring again to *The Sports Gene* book by David Epstein, he pointed out that major league baseball players are able to hit a 90-mph fast pitch because their brain does what is called "chunking." That is, the brain remembering seeing that pitch over and over again until the brain only needs to see the beginning of the pitch to know where the ball is headed.

We need to do the same thing in karate, see thousands of live reverse punches (not choreographed stepping forward lunge punches), and know by the movement of the opponents' hips what is coming.

To build this chunking in your brain is to perform repetitive drills, as athletes with more experience tend to have better timing. Being able to anticipate events by 'reading the movement' often gained through experience allows the kumite player to demonstrate good timing because they get into the correct position early. An athlete with better timing will be able to perform at a quicker rate. There are no tests available for timing, but you know it when you see it, or feel it.

You can certainly create your own timing drills but to get you started try this simple drill. Get a tether ball, you know the ball on a rope. Have a partner swing the ball around in circles over their head so that it swings around their body. Try and time the ball and score on their body without getting hit. Also, get back out of the circle of the ball before it hits you. This forces you to think about timing and distance and move quickly-just like you're in a match.

In order to improve your ability to fight at a distance, we need to improve our depth perception and peripheral vision. This is your distance radar, just like in the old movies when the submarine got closer and closer, we watched the dot on the screen move ominously closer. Your eyes and brain integrate and tell you when you opponent is in range. Fighters are continuously moving in and out of great striking range. It happens all match long. The first one to recognize the appropriate distance usually wins. Therefore, one method to consider during a conditioning circuit is to have one attacker (tori) throw reverse punches at head level, for a defined amount of time, trying to set up and score, while tori (the one receiving the initial technique) has to split the timing with a counter reverse punch to the body. This can actually be more productive than sparring because there typically aren't clashes and there are much fewer injuries. By using the opposing strike heights possibility of hand slamming into each other is eliminated as well. This would make for a great station in a conditioning circuit. Many variations can similarly be devised as well.

CONSIDERATION #4 THE PHYSIOLOGICAL TRAIT OF BALANCE

Proper balance is important in unlocking your full athletic potential and can quickly help you become a more stable attacker, smoother at pivoting, better at aiming, throwing, and kicking, while lowering risk of injury.

This makes sense when you notice most movement and striking techniques you must go through a transition off one leg, and rapidly onto the other in perfect balance, often times while being potentially knocked off balance by a moving opponent. For example, think about a simple front kick, mae-geri, which involves the transference of weight from one leg to the other, with one leg firmly planting and the other swinging into a kick.

Why worry about balance in karate conditioning? Because our modern lifestyle is dealing a serious blow to the human balance system. In primitive times, our balance was constantly challenged by the uneven ground and varied terrain that we traveled every day. Now, we move in a world designed to protect us from falls—smooth, even sidewalks, exceptionally flat floors, perfectly proportional stairs, and shoes worn sixteen hours a day that help stabilize the feet. Nowadays a crack in the pavement is cause for complaints and yellow tape to warn us away from the hazard. Perfectly aligned living and workspaces are not the only causes of our balance loss. You can add electronic digital screens, universally poor shoe design, archaic fitness methods, and even eyeglasses as contributing factors to humans evolving with less balance.

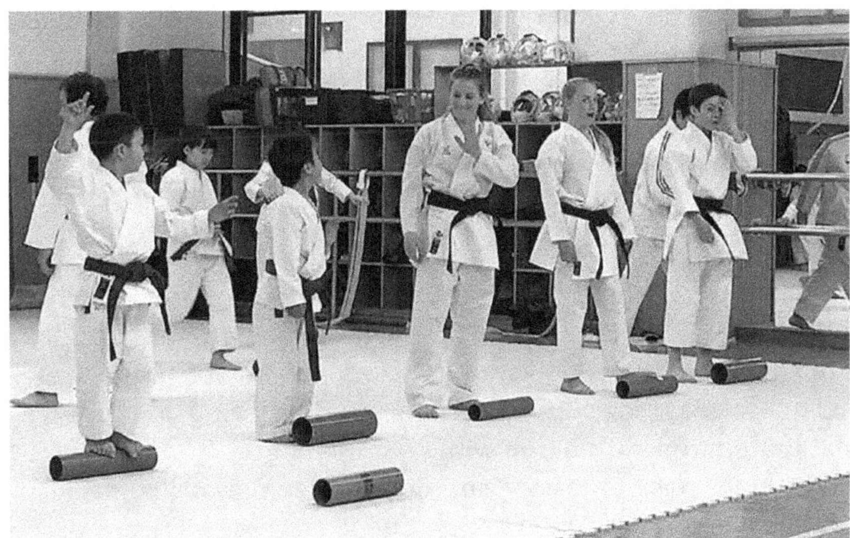

Balance Training in Japan

Restoring our natural potential, or possibly attaining maximal balance isn't exclusively reliant upon building new muscles or developing new skills. It is not about, as the saying goes, teaching an old dog new tricks. In fact, it is difficult to describe how rapidly the body resets its sense of balance without invoking the word magic. The fact is, with minimal effort, the body's balance system has a way of simply rebooting itself.

It has been stated previously in this chapter you should develop your own training drills to meet your needs, but here are a few thoughts on drills for consideration.

One-Legged Balance

Start with this beginning move, keeping a stable chair or a wall within arms' reach. With feet together, pick up one foot—knee facing forward or to the side. Hold the position for thirty seconds with eyes open, then closed. Then do it while turning your lead sideways to the left and right. Switch feet and repeat for the same number of reps on each foot. You can stand on one leg and execute a mae-geri, and then yoko-geri followed by ushiro-geri. Once this is easy, consider a move to standing on a wooden 2"x4" board.

One-Legged Clock with Arms

Balance on one leg, torso straight, head up, and hands on the hips. Visualize a clock and point your arm straight overhead to 12, then to the side (three), and then circle low and around to nine without losing your balance.

Increase the challenge by having a partner call out the different times to you. Switch to the opposite arm and leg and repeat.

Clock on an Unstable Surface

Once you master balance moves on solid ground, try them on an unstable surface such as a Bosu ball, Dyna Disc, Wobble Board, Airex Pad, or balance plank. Some studies have suggested that training on an unstable surface does not ensure that balance will improve when performing on a stable surface, but at worst, you might strengthen the lower leg stabilizers and have a fun variation in training that promotes compliance.

Like all of the aforementioned drills/concepts, these can be incorporated into rest intervals during the rounds in the circuit, or between circuits.

One-Legged Squat

Stand with your feet hip-width apart. Point your left foot out front, just barely touching the floor for balance and push your hips back and down into this challenging one-legged squat position. Your right knee is bent, chest upright, eyes forward, and your arms out front. Slowly push up to return to starting position. Switch feet. Be sure the knee doesn't push in front of the toes. Once you master this flat footed, repeat the drill with your heel of the ground on your support leg. This is actually a truer "athletic position," since appropriate locomotion in most all of sport is done on the toes and not with the heels resting on the ground.

Single-Leg Romanian Dead Lift

Balance on your left foot, engage the entire core, front, side and back, and bend forward at the hips while reaching toward the ground with your right hand. Hold on to a weight and raise your right leg behind you for counterbalance. Maintain a neutral spine. Tighten the buttocks as you return to the starting position. Keep your knee relaxed and back flat throughout the movement. Switch legs.

One last comment on balance: **Balance exercises should be done in a controlled environment that stimulates your sense of balance while minimizing risk. This idea is called "controlled instability." Drills like doing heavy squats while balancing precariously on a physio ball are not recommended.**

ANALYZING AND ENCORPORATING THE PSYCHO-PHYSIOLOGY FACTORS WHICH CONTRIBUTE TO KUMITE SUCCESS

Now that we have considered physiological traits peculiar to our unique physiology, it's time to investigate psycho-physiological traits (skills affecting the physiological response as a result of the psyche.)

Below are some principles that include a mental component in moving during a match. This may seem like minutia in designing a fitness component but often times, great matches are won by minutia. They suggest some technical/tactical issues for your consideration in choosing what to include in the conditioning program/circuit, as a means towards greater overall performance.

The ideal traits and desired outcomes are:

1. **Be Present:** The focus is on the present, no thoughts of the future or past. Can you turn on and off in focus immediately, or are you a prisoner to your own mind? This ability to be present can be trained.
2. **Movement:** The ability to move in all directions, to get you in to score or out of trouble. can be trained.
3. **Preparation to score:** Unless you are faster than every opponent you will need to have ability to set up and pull off scoring attacks. You must also have the confidence to do so. This can be trained.
4. **Explosive movement:** When you move you must commit yourself full speed without doubt. This can be trained.
5. **Execution:** Your techniques should be mechanically sound. This can be trained.
6. **Recovery:** after you attack, regardless of if you scored or not, you are not finished. You may have to retreat or move laterally. This can be trained.

The best way to inculcate these principles is to incorporate them into your training during skill acquisition time. When you pick a drill or develop a drill go over each principle to keep it in mind as you train. Once you've mastered the skill and can repeat it continuously, it can be included in the conditioning component of practice, if desired.

PSYCHO-PHYSIOLOGICAL PRINCIPLE #1: BEING PRESENT

One method of maintaining presence before you enter the enter the ring is to center your mind. You can learn to do this through relaxation techniques and belly breathing, which is inhaling for four seconds and exhaling for four seconds, while expanding the belly outwards. Attention should be given so that the breathing isn't done with the rib cage traveling vertically, up, and down. Proper belly breathing puts the body in a parasympathetic state (relaxed), and not a sympathetic state of anxiety. This is obviously important in creating the mushin ("no mind") state that fighters seek. When you do so, remind yourself this is to center your attention, with no thoughts of previous competition, or the future. Only now exists. Part of being present is to stay alert.

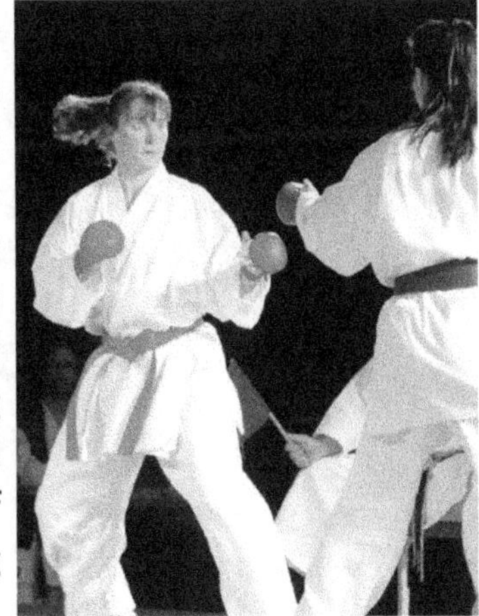

To be present you must learn to stay in the moment, you want to be completely focused on the task at hand. Where you place your attention matters because that is where your energy is directed. Do not think of the past, only think of this moment.

Staying in the present and remaining alert is not as easy as it sounds. If you think about driving a car, you will say you must be alert and pay attention. But most car accidents happen when the driver is distracted, engaging in a conversation with other passengers in the car, making or receiving phone calls, sending, or receiving text messages, eating while driving or events outside the car may cause driver distraction. But if you ask the driver if they are paying attention, they likely say, "yes."

Staying present and alert, takes skill and practice. The first step is to be cognitve of the effort.

When doing drills to clear out your mind, focus on the drill, telling yourself there is no past, no future, only now. These can be done for 10-15 seconds between circuit exercises, as a station in the circuit, or between rounds of the circuit.

Whether you're in training and focusing on a drill or in the middle of competition, do not think about outcome-only process. To paraphrase the great coach John Wooden, "satisfaction comes from the knowledge of knowing you did your best." That means focus on the process of training or focus on the process of competition. Doing so many big things and little things properly id incredibly hard on its own. There is no room for diverting your focus to outcome. If you do, you aren't doing the process right.

World Champion boxer "Sugar" Ray Leonard said when he was present and alert, his eyes got as big as silver dollars. With him there was no past, and no future. There was only the present, the way it should be when you're continually fighters trained killers like Roberto Duran, Thomas Hearns and Marvin Hagler, Hector Camacho, and Wilfred Benitez.

The rest intervals between rounds of the circuit would be a perfect time to practice deep belly breathing and attaining a state of an empty mind. It would also make a nice post-circuit cool down. A much more detailed explanation of this will be found later in this book in the "Mental Programming" section.

PSYCHO-PHYSIOLOGICAL PRINCIPLE #2: MOVEMENT

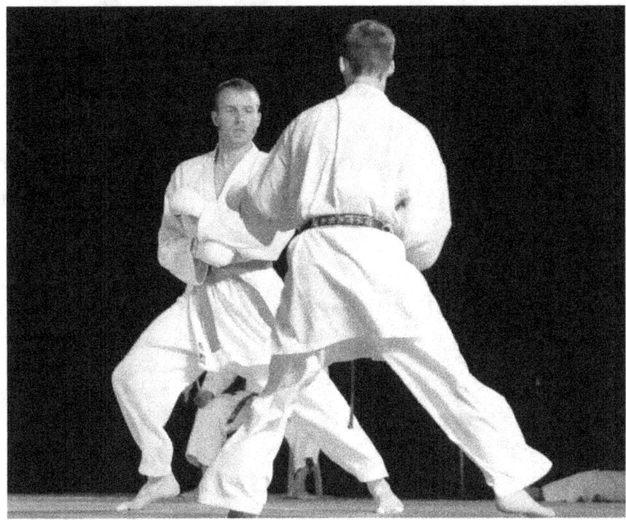

It is best to control your opponent, not to have all of your movements be a reaction to theirs. You can control the ring with movement. Everything good comes from your movement. Your goal should be to be your best moving version of you that you can be, moving forward, backwards, and laterally. Change of direction is of paramount importance. Failure to believe in your movement ability can be somewhat paralyzing, and you cannot win that way.

The simplest drill:

Shuffle forward, then back, then left then right. Include this in attacking or countering. Once you master this as a solo drill, do it in response to a visual stimulus. You can create many more, incorporating an uke, various objects such as thrown balls, or heavy bags to counter punch/ kick after your movement, or other creations. YouTube will have a wealth of information on how the world's best do it.

Focus on movement of the feet one at a time. Do some drills when you are fresh to develop the skills needed. Then start to move faster and faster. When you are technically proficient at fast speeds, they can be included in the conditioning part of the daily program. It's a double win this way: the conditioning gets better and the karate gets better

PSYCHO-PHYSIOLOGICAL PRINCIPLE #3: PREPARING TO SCORE

In your drills, and in competition, you should always set up your attack or counter. For example, if you prefer to counter, you should consider moving forward to draw the opponent's attack. At higher levels, this works better than the novice protocol of stepping back, blocking, and then countering. It is a favorite technique of Seiji Nishimura. If you prefer to attack, work on different set-ups from which to throw the same best scoring technique. These drills should be perfected at slow speeds during a time when you're fresh. As you progress with sound technique, increase speed. When they become habits and are in good technique, they are ready for inclusion into the conditioning component of the total daily and weekly plan. Improvement in movement abilities will help the athlete to move more efficiently and successfully and a corresponding confidence in such will accompany it.

PSYCHO-PHYSIOLOGICAL PRINCIPLE #4: EXPLOSIVE MOVEMENT

Once you are committed to your attack, you must explode. You should also do this on the counterattack, no half measures. The same as applies to your evasion, your blocking and your feinting. Explosion separates champions from non-winners in most every sport. Karate is no exception. Explosive movement starts with the nervous system trying to fire immediately, and calling upon more signals to fire, and to continue to recruit more fast twitch fibers to contract. This is called rate coding.

Always spend a great amount of your time practicing technique of new movements at a slower pace until you've engrained great biomechanics. Don't rush the process. Focus on your process here. Once it is a very refined and repeatable skill you have to throw techniques at full speed, with lots of rest. You cannot get fast throwing slow techniques. It's impossible.

Working diligently on this over the course of years can make a huge change in performance, which is why most high school athletes and all college, professional and Olympic athletes devote extreme amounts of training time towards acquiring this trait. Indeed, speed kills, and speed can be significantly improved through proper strength training methods. That is why virtually all world class sprinters on land, in water or on ice pursue vigorous strength training programs. This is critical to success.

PSYCHO-PHYSIOLOGICAL PRINCIPLE #5: EXECUTION

Execution all of your work up to this point will be wasted if you do not execute the technique properly. The technique must be clean, posture appropriate and strong, devoid of extraneous movement. It is important to know that conditioning circuits are not a good place to try to enhance this trait. The body is simply too fatigued.

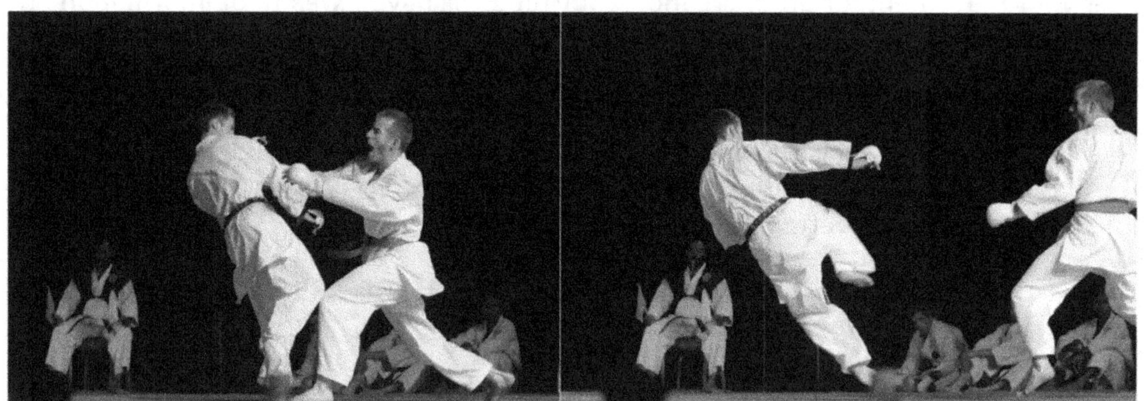

PSYCHO-PHYSIOLOGICAL PRINCIPLE #6: RECOVERY

After you score, you must recover and break off the engagement distance to prevent a counter score or your opponent hitting you. This can be either a lateral movement or retreating movement. Great fighters can do both. This is something too many karate players struggle with, likely the cause of spending most of their training time moving forward in blitzing and/or devoting an inordinate amount of time to drilling basic mechanical movements, which have already been engrained for years or decades.

The fix here is simple. Spend time moving in recovery patterns you wish to improve. These can certainly be included in conditioning circuits once the skill is engrained with good mechanics. Using resisted cords can be very valuable in promoting strength and power gains, while increasing the heart rate and the conditioning effect.

The fact is, with these psycho-physiological considerations if an athlete believes they can't, they won't. If they believe they can, they have a much better chance at pulling that off. Drills to target specific areas, will increase of a successful outcome in athletes. We always want fighters to believe that they can.

THE PHILOSOPHY GOVERNING ELITE PERFORMER'S CIRCUIT CONSTRUCTION

Now that we have covered the most important part of on-mat conditioning (how to make conditioning specific to your karate,) we can discuss how to construct the circuits for elite competitors to make them most beneficial.

There are many factors to manipulate in circuit design, such as choice of exercises, duration of exercise, total volume of work to be performed, length of rest intervals, number of circuits to be performed, number of exercises, recovery between stations, order of exercises and rest between rounds. All must point towards performance optimization for those training to be elite, and performance enhancement and increased fitness for non-competitors.

The overall philosophy that should govern circuit creation is that the goal is to optimize an athlete's karate-specific fitness demands safely and efficiently for use in elite competition.

This is karate. This is a combat sport, where only the toughest survive. This is conditioning day.

To be prepared for a "survival of the fittest challenge", you have to have elite fitness, and that should never be compromised.

Boxing legend Muhammad Ali said, "The fight is won or lost far away from the witnesses, behind the lines, in the gym and out there on the road." This is pretty much a universally accepted philosophy in boxing, as personal conversations with coaches of world champion fighters revealed that their goal is to be in great shape for 125 percent of the fight demands. This means that a young pro fighting three-minute rounds should be fit enough to spar four-minute rounds. It also means those fighting in eight round fights should be capable of fighting ten solid rounds. Again, this must be done safely, without overtraining, but an athlete who is serious about competition should get close to that state.

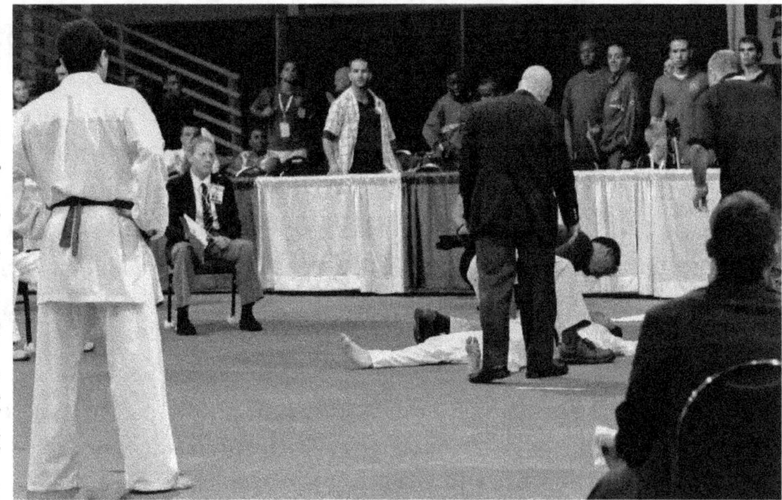

A good way to look at this philosophically would be through use of the Heart Rate Zones Model. Simply stated, a person can achieve a training heart rate that can be divided into one of five zones. The best way to find your heart rate is to use a heart rate monitor. Simply run very hard up a long hill and see how high you can get it. If you don't have the monitor, run that same hill as hard as you can and then take your pulse for fifteen seconds. Multiply that number times four. Or, if you're more comfort seeking, subtract your age from the number 220 for an acceptable estimate. If the heart rate is fairly low in exercise, between fifty to sixty percent on one's maximum heart rate (MHR), they are in zone one. This is purely aerobic (oxidative) and relies primarily upon breakdown of fats. This really isn't specific to karate and not very useful in the training. Zone two is the place where the percentage of MRH is sixty to seventy percent. Zone three are the heart rates between seventy and eighty percent, zone four ranges from eighty to ninety percent. The Grand Daddy of them all is zone five. This is where heart rates soar to between ninety to one hundred percent. If running, for example, zone one would be a brisk walk or slow jog, zone two a jog, zone three a jog in a hilly area, zone four a hard run and zone five, a sprint like the 400 meters. In the dojo it might look like this: zone one movements are easy warming up drills, zone two might be doing "rice line" kihon movements, throwing techniques while moving up and down the floor, zone three being sparring drills at a sweat-breaking pace, zone four being like sparring drills or fighting rounds against lesser opponents and zone five is like being in high action wars in National or International Tournaments.

The conditioning circuit should not be easy. Matches aren't easy. The energy demands in a match can be taxing. Therefore, there should be a lot of training time spent in zones four and five, just as there can be in matches. This isn't to say that the entire time should be spent there. There are times in matches where the pace slows down and fighters regroup. Rather, there should be very fatiguing stations where the heart rate hits zone five and is there for some time, perhaps followed by an easier station that drops it back down into zone two or three. An example might be a thirty second station of resisted split squat jumps, followed by a thirty second station of resisted cord blitzing, followed by a thirty second bout of defending attacks of an attacker that is throwing techniques continuously. This would elicit a heart rate response in zone five and might be followed by a station of focused vision training, such as balancing on one leg and doing a depth perception drill. The number of circuits one can design are infinite, and circuits must be changed very often to alleviate staleness both physically and mentally.

To elicit this rapid and intense heart rate response total body, full exertional movements, like dumbbell split squat jumps, pull-ups, dips, step-ups, lunge variations, hill sprints, pedaling a resisted bike, resisted cord attacks, shuttle runs, defending against fresh partners, or attacking against someone continuously who only defends. There should also be some drills that are not quite as intense, to keep a heart rate in a high zone but not too high, like lateral movement drills, footwork drills, or hitting a speed bag. Finally, there can be recovery exercises, like deep belly breathing, focus training, vision training, or even walking laps around the floor. It's important to be creative. Incorporate sport-specific, or individual-specific movements for skill execution under a state of sympathetic stress in the body.

Since matches last one and a half minutes for youth, and up to three minutes for elite adults, you will need to have the competitor fit enough to exert themselves that long, or if you follow the lead of the elite boxing coaches, perhaps four hard minutes would be a worthy goal. Some circuits should therefore be three or four minutes long. Four rounds of that with a significant rest between rounds would be an exceptional conditioning day and would provide many significant adaptations in a fighter's physiology.

Obviously, it would be exceptionally rare to maintain a heart rate in zone five that entire time, but that doesn't happen in a match anyway. Remember, karate is sport of exploding, and slowing down to implement strategy. The athlete will have huge heart rate fluctuations in matches, and we need to have them prepared for that.

Another way to enhance fitness would be to create shorter circuits, that are even more intense, such as doing eight two-minute rounds, with a two-minute rest. The goal here would be to hit zone five as fast as possible and maintain it until the round ends. Then during the rest interval relax and lower the heart rate as much as possible. Conversely, longer, less intense circuits can be devised, such as three rounds of eight minutes where less intense exercises are prescribed and lower heart rates, like zone three, are maintained throughout the round.

There are many different methods of ordering the exercises, such as alternating exercises that are predominantly upper body movements with lower body movements, alternating one strength/endurance resistance exercise like kettlebell swings with two karate specific exercise, like one attacking while in resisted cords and the other defending against the resisted cord attacker. Many formats are possible. Create one to meet your needs.

The beauty of this system is continual new stimulus psychologically, continual new stimulus for body adaptations, it's sport-specific or individual specific, weaknesses in karate ability or physiology (such as vision or lagging lateral movement ability) can be addressed and corrected and it only takes about thirty minutes to complete. This is an exceptionally productive and efficient protocol. Examples might be constructed to look like this:

FIGURE 57:

DAY 1:

4 MINUTE CIRCUIT for an attacking fighter

Perform each station for 30 seconds, with a three-minute rest between rounds. Do 3 rounds.

1. Ten-yard shuttle run

2. Resisted cord blitzing

3. Defending in corner against uke attacking non-stop

4. Dumbbell Squat Jumps

5. Plank Hold

6. Individual Footwork Drill

7. Split Squat Jumps

8. Shadow kumite against an opponent who remains 10 meters away

This consists of (7) 30 second stations, which seems like it won't take four minutes, but there is time between stations to get the athlete to the next station. This is a very hard circuit and affords the participant to significantly enhance their conditioning and lactate threshold, while using some sport-specific drills to enhance carryover to match performance.

Another example of a session might be:

FIGURE 58:

DAY 2:

2 MINUTE CIRCUIT for an attacking fighter

Circuit A: Perform each station for 30 seconds, with a minute rest between rounds. Do 2 rounds.

1. Resisted Cord Lateral Hops

2. Heavy Bag Combinations (jab-reverse-roundhouse) as many as possible

3. Repeat Side Hops over an ace wrap

4. Kumite, defending only, no attacking

Circuit B: Perform each station for 30 seconds, with a minute rest between rounds. Do 2 rounds.

1. Resisted Cord Retreating

2. Kettlebell Swings

3. Clapping Push-ups

4. Split Squat Jumps

Virtually thousands of exercises/drills can be inserted into the circuit and millions of combinations are possible. Circuits can include running if desired, or methods not typically utilized in dojos, such as row machines, strongman events like the farmer's carry, judo exercises or anything else that can stimulate the participant.

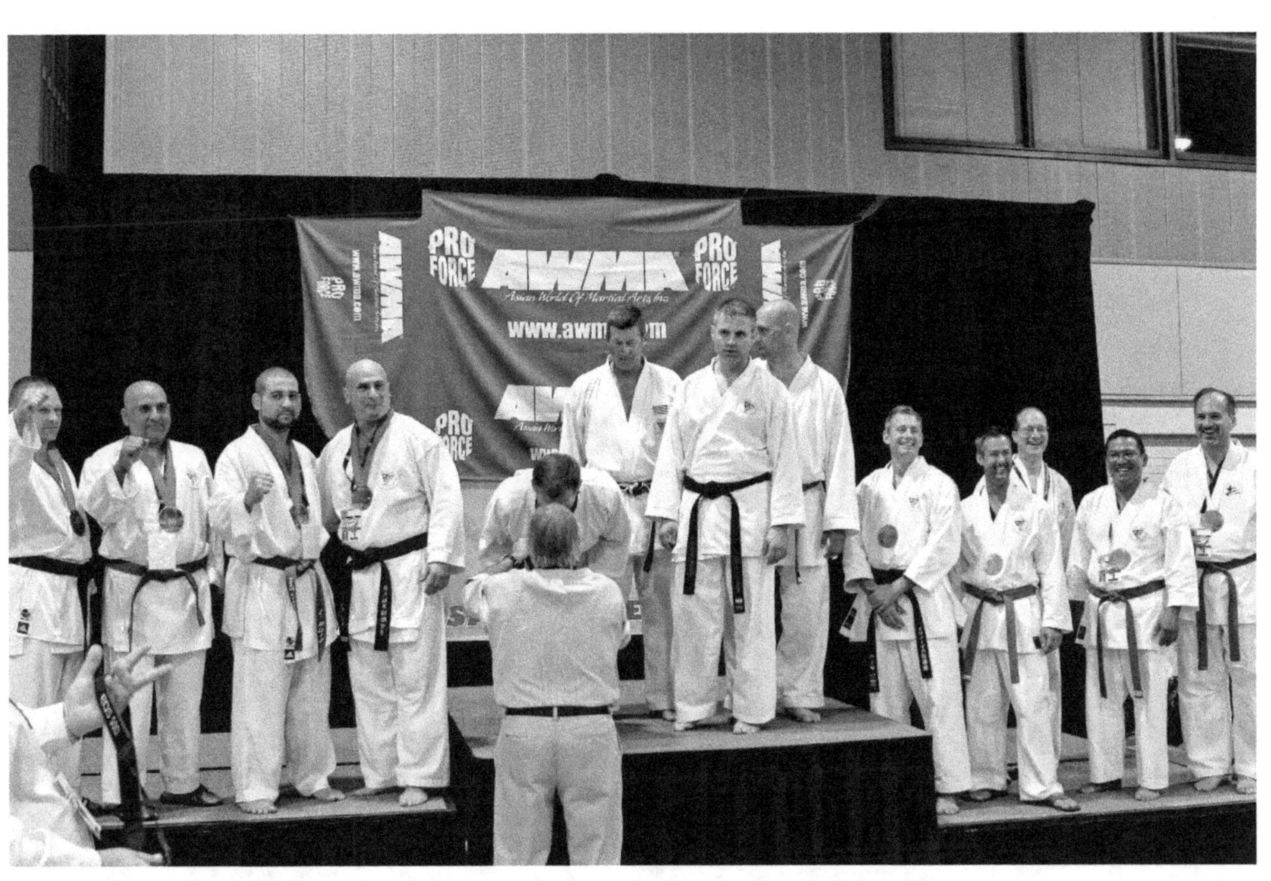
PRO FORCE
AWMA
Asian World Of Martial Arts Inc
www.awma.com
PRO FORCE

5
Warm-Ups

No weightlifter wants to attempt a personal record clean and jerk without being fully warmed up and prepared. No sprinter competes in an all-out race effort without warming up. No pitcher throws his fastest fast ball without extreme diligence in warming up. Karate athletes should never throw a jodan mawashi-geri, or any technique for that matter, without an appropriate warm up.

Warming up is a commonality to all athletes, regardless of the physiological differences of their competitive endeavor. But what exactly is a "proper" or "great" warm-up? What have the last hundred years of millions of athletes world-wide that did warm-ups have to teach us today? What does science teach us?

We have no definitive answer on the ideal warm-up. Decades ago, pure calisthenics, like jumping jacks, torso rotations and windmill toe touches were the preferred protocol. That was morphed into a system that primarily consisted of static stretching. Coaches and athletes then realized that static stretching was productive in increasing passive range of motion about a joint, but wasn't optimal in promoting ideal mobility (active, dynamic range of motion) or in increasing body temperature and synovial fluid release. The trend thus became a warm-up consisting exclusively or primarily of mobility exercises, which were essentially moving stretches, like knee-to-chest walks, or straight leg lunges walks, etc. It was at this time that the thought prevailed that because moving stretches (mobility exercises) were good, that static stretching was bad. Many coaches and athletes quit doing static stretches and lost the benefits they offered. And interestingly enough, while these were the trends in the exercise scientists were prescribing, and many athletes were doing, there was a huge diversity among cultures. The weightlifters were not doing the mobility exercises the way the track sprinters were. They were using wooden rods and performing movements such as shoulder mobility circles, torso rotations, good morning, and squat range of motion exercises. This is drastically different than what swimmers were doing, and track athletes, and professional baseball pitchers.

Practical experience has also provided interesting anecdotal information. In the boxing gym a program of shadow boxing and rope jumping was the daily introduction to the work-out. In a judo dojo, warm-up (junbi undo) consisted exclusively of tandoku renshu (mimicking throws moving in various directions, such as forward, backwards, sideways and at diagonals, without a partner). There was never one stretch performed over two decades and there was never a tweaked muscle. That goes against all odds predicted by our sports scientists. This protocol differed greatly from the Wado-Ryu karate dojo, which differed from the Shotokan karate dojo, which differed greatly from the ones administered in our local competition team practice that produced many National Champions. In fact, at a renowned clinic is Park City, Utah, we once delivered a highly sport-specific movement protocol established exclusively for karate. It consisted of movements specific to the sport in increasing intensity of difficulty. At first, 5 easy lead hand punches with each arm were thrown. Then five reverse punches were thrown. Next was five easy combinations of the two, followed by backfists. Bent knee raises, front kicks slowly thrown, side leg hip abductions and sidekicks were also gently performed. This escalated in complexity and intensity. It was akin to tandoku renshu and much science was presented to support the practice of this protocol. This was used very successfully in a team that won many national championships as a team, and as individuals. It seemed very conclusive, but as fate would have it, the next clinician in the following presentation led the class through a warm-up that had nothing to do with the preceding one. That instructor had not attended the previous clinic presentation and led a warm-up very contrary to it. But, in his defense, he was an exceptional practitioner, exceptional teacher and an exceptional leader whose students had no history of pulled muscles. He obviously was not "wrong" in his approach, as evidenced by his track record. It was an interesting life experience. So, which one is right, and which is wrong?

The sport scientists of today all seem to concur that a proper warm-up/stretching/mobility/activation protocol will provide the following physiological adaptations: temperature increases in the muscle, which lead to strength and speed enhancements, blood temperature increases which enables increases the amount of oxygen the bold holds, increased range of motion about the joints, decreased potential for muscle tears, decreased awkward and inefficient movement which can decrease performance and increase risk of injury, not to mention psychological preparedness and a sense of readiness and well-being.

Therefore, athletes should continue to warm-up daily and view this period of time as being every bit as valuable as the heart of the practice itself. Here are a few current thoughts for the karateka in this period of practice.

The National Strength and Conditioning Association is recognized as a premier authority in the preparation of athletes for performance. They prescribe a "R.A.M.P." program, which consists of:

R: Raise. Raise the temperature of the muscles and blood through mild aerobic exercise, like jogging, riding a bicycle or jumping a rope.
A: Activate. Activate the muscles through easy bodyweight exercises that force the muscles to contract, such as bodyweight squats, lunges, or push-ups.
M: Mobilize. Move the muscles that will be needed in practice or competition through increase range of motion, by doing active movements through increasing end ranges.
P: Potentiate. Perform movements such as squat jumps or low level plyometrics to force a rapid recruitment of fibers.

The National Association of Sports Medicine offers a corrective exercise protocol that many strength and conditioning coaches have adapted for their "warm-up/pre-hab/activation" prescription. Their adapted structure of this model can be as follows:

1. **Inhibition:** Inhibit the tension in the muscles through use of foam rolling, massage of even mechanical massage machine use.
2. **Lengthening.** This would be a time for the preferred active mobility patterns and can also incorporate some static stretching if the athlete feels this modality can increase their preparedness.
3. **Isolate.** Perform a non-complex, simple movement to isolate a muscle and insure that is firing properly.
4. **Integrate.** Perform more complex movements that are more sport-specific, like diagonal lunges.

Another interesting concept worthy of consideration was designed by Cal Dietz and associates in their Reflexive Performance Rest protocol. In this method, after an athletic warm-up protocol athletes are instructed through a series of vigorous self-massaging points on trigger points, thought to promote activation in sending neurological impulses to muscles that may not be actively firing at optimal levels. Dietz performs a series of manual isometric tests to assess if muscles are indeed firing. If they aren't firing instantly, he or the athlete rubs the corresponding trigger point (which is elsewhere in the body) and it seems to activate the previously sluggish or non-responsive muscles group. Many practitioners exposed to this swear by it, making claims that it can even enhance an athlete's speed or reduce team injury levels significantly.

Regardless of the chosen protocol, a few commonalities probably exist worthy of consideration in the design and implementation of the warm-up protocol:

1. The well-being and feeling of being fully prepared is important to the performance of the athlete. Almost all athletes get this feeling from rolling out on foam rollers or balls, like basketballs or volleyballs. This is worthy of time in most cases.
2. Increasing temperature of the muscles and blood is recognized by most as an essential practice. Performing lower intensity exercises to "break a sweat" would seem to be a valid recommendation.
3. Moving stretches, such as knee-to-chest pulls, inchworm walks, walking straight leg lunges and additional patterns are universally used worldwide by track and field athletes that are at the pinnacle of speed and power development, two traits required to be successful in most sports, including karate.
4. Static stretching is not a tool of evil, and some athletes feel more confident incorporating it. Perhaps a minute or two can be designated as a period of self-prescription so that athletes can buy into the program more because they own part of the decision making.
5. Activation into more sport specific movements seems to be essential. Think back to the aforementioned examples at the judo dojo (tandoku renshu), the shadow boxing, the karate clinic and the activation or integration sought by the NSCA and NASM. This could be a time for an athlete to choose a movement pattern they're struggling with, such as lateral movement in response to a front kick, and work this slowly and correctly to engrain it, before moving to faster speeds. This would also provide the athlete with the above mentioned "ownership" of their performance needs and outcome. This could also be a place to plug in kata practice for the traditional approach of performing both kata and kumite in the dojo.

FIGURE 59:

A sample non-specific/general warm-up program can be designed like this:

1. JOG: 5 minutes

2. FOAM ROLL: 30 seconds each:

    a. L calf

    b. R calf

    c. L hamstring

    d. R hamstring

    e. L glute

    f. R glute

    g. L IT band

    h. R IT band

    i. L quad

    j. R quad

    k. L groin

    l. R groin

3. YOGA STRETCHES: 30-60 seconds each

    a. Child's pose

    b. Cobra

    c. Downward dog

    d. L Leg Forward Pigeon

    e. R Leg Forward Pigeon

    f. L Leg half Kneeling Hip Flexor

    g. R Leg half Kneeling Hip Flexor

    h. Butterfly pulling on Feet

    i. Butterfly Elbows on Knees

    j. L Side Lying Quad

    k. R Side Lying Quad

    l. L Calf

    m. R Calf

FIGURE 60:

A sample karate-specific warm-up program can therefore be constructed such as this:

RAISE/ACTIVATE

1. 5 Each (at any easy speed, with no rest between exercises):
    a. Jab
    b. Reverse Punch
    c. Jab-Reverse Combination
    d. Front Kick
    e. Lead Leg Roundhouse kick
    f. Back Leg Roundhouse kick
    g. Sidekick
    h. Shift back, Block and Counter

MOBILIZE

2. Mobility Movements (approximately 10 yards each):
    a. Marching on Toes
    b. Knee to Chest Walk
    c. Leg Cradles
    d. Quads
    e. Backwards hamstring
    f. Quad with RDL
    g. Lateral Groin – both directions
    h. Cross Over Toe Touch
    i. Kicks
    j. Twisting Lunges

POTENTIATE

3. 5 Each:
    a. Squat Jumps
    b. Split Squat Jumps
    c. Push-up
4. 30 seconds Kumite Shadow Sparring at 80% speed

FEELING OF PREPAREDNESS/OWNERSHIP TIME

5. 1 minute of self-selected stretching

POTENTIATE

6. 30 seconds full speed Kumite Shadow Sparring

Another example could be:

FIGURE 61:

INHIBIT

1. FOAM ROLL: 30 seconds each:
   a. L calf
   b. R calf
   c. L hamstring
   d. R hamstring
   e. L glute
   f. R glute
   g. L IT band
   h. R IT band
   i. L quad
   j. R quad
   k. L groin
   l. R groin

ACTIVATE

2. Pick a movement pattern (such as a blitz, lateral movement, defensive footwork, transition from defense to offense, etc.): 5 minutes on own, starting slow and increasing in speed and intensity until a sweat is broken.

LENGTHEN/MOBILIZE

3. Mobility Movements (approximately 10 yards each):
   a. Marching on Toes
   b. Knee to Chest Walk
   c. Leg Cradles
   d. Quads
   e. Backwards hamstring
   f. Quad with RDL
   g. Lateral Groin – both directions
   h. Cross Over Toe Touch
   i. Kicks
   j. Twisting Lunges

There are virtually endless possibilities that an instructor/coach or athlete can design, and programs should be changed frequently to alleviate both psychological and physiological staleness.

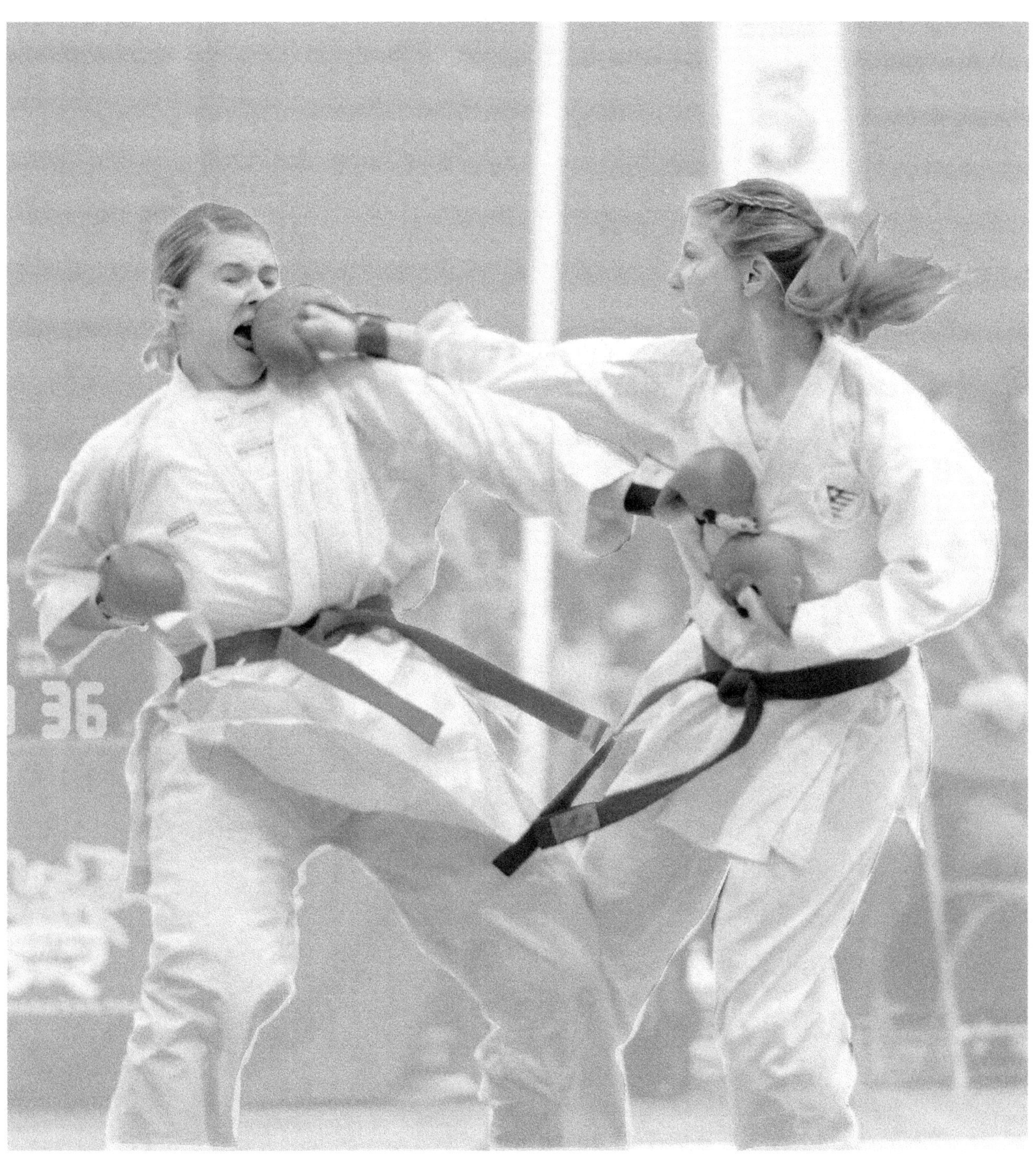

6

Mental
Programming

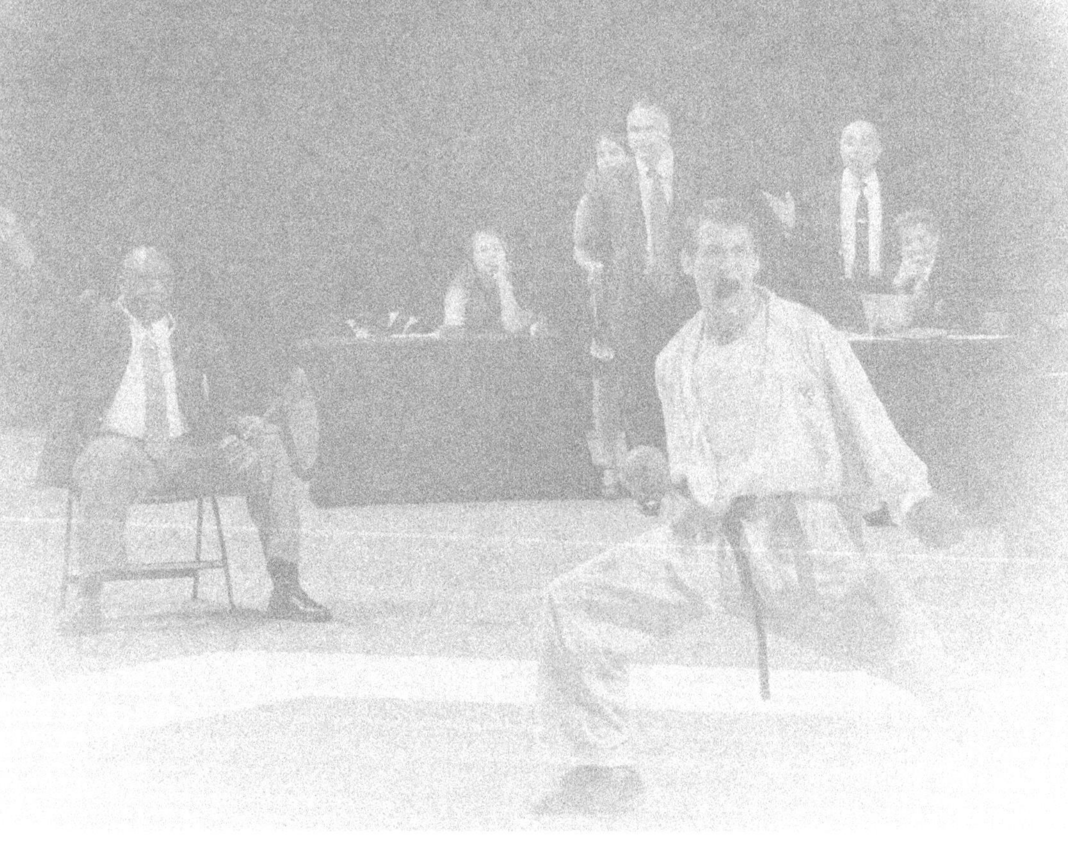

INTRODUCTION

For many decades we have been asking athletes, "what percentage of your sport is mental" Invariably the response is an unusually high number, typically 70 percent or higher. Sometimes we even hear 100 percent, an impossibility. Regardless, the over whelming feeling is that most athletes believe there is a significant contribution from the mental side. The next question we ask is how much time athletes devote intentionally to mental training. That's where we get blank stares, and the proverbial "aha" light bulb shines above their heads. They realize that they are severely neglecting the area they feel most contributes to their performance. To facilitate a better "mental game," this next section has been designed as an interactive workbook. It starts with a basic understanding of the benefits of mental training and progresses into goal setting, visualization, and other advanced techniques.

STEP 1: ACKNOWLEDGE THE POWER OF THE MIND THROUGH UNDERSTANDING HOW IT FUNCTIONS

Put the following FACTS forefront in your heart and mind. These facts can significantly change your vision, performance outcome and your life!

- Your mind acts just like a computer. Whatever is programmed into it, is what it acts upon.

- The law of computers says, "garbage in equals garbage out." If you put good things in the computer, you will get good out of it. Likewise, negative inputs yield negative outputs. For example, if you program into your computer 2 + 2 = 5 (bad input), every time you add 2 + 2, you will get the wrong answer. However, if you program 2 + 2 =4 (good input), you will get the correct answer every time. The brain works much like this. If you continually bombard the brain with negative thoughts, it will tend to act out on them and provide that outcome.

- Your mind also works much the way a man drives a car. The man in the car is like the conscious mind. It is a small part of the total mass, but a valuable part. He deciphers what he sees as truths (where to steer, the appropriate driving speed, when to brake, etc.) The bulk of the car (body), like the bulk of the brain, is like the subconscious mind. Its job is to act out on the viewpoint of the driver and to perform. All it does is act on input and get that job done it is programmed to do. The gas pedal is your self-belief. If you believe strongly, you are "pedal to the metal, full speed ahead," and capable of winning the race. If you doubt yourself, you are idling.

- Your brain is therefore programmed. It is programmed by your thoughts, words, and past experiences.

- It is CRITICAL to continually flood your brain with positive affirmations and visualizations of success. This programs your computer positively and gives it good directions to act out upon.

- An athlete cannot out-perform their self-image. The man (or woman) who thinks he can and the man (or woman) who thinks he can't are both right.

- Self-talk on average, is approximately a staggering 77% negative. That means, the average person is programming negative thoughts into their computer (brain) almost 80% of the time. This is what the mind has to act upon. Garbage in equals garbage out. The subconscious mind acts on the negative input and follows blindly. This causes negative results in performance.

- Research studies indicate that schoolteacher's negative feedback to students (mind programming) is often over half of the total feedback, while coaches provided over 75% negative feedbacks. This can severely damage an athlete's performance.

- The Mayo Clinic identifies four types of negative self-talk:

  1. Filtering is where you focus on the negative. Scenario: you gained a pound this week and you focus on this and ignore the fact that you have already lost 25 pounds.

  2. Personalizing is where you feel everything is your fault. Scenario: your training partner cancels out on a training session with you due to a nagging injury, but you feel it is because of you.

  3. Catastrophizing is the fear the worst will always happen. Scenario: You cannot beat the opponent in front of you because they are always bigger, stronger, faster, or more talented than you in your mind, or their kicks in warm-ups looked better than you perceive yours to be.

  4. Polarizing is the feeling that you must always be perfect. Scenario: your legs felt heavy in warmups so you think you cannot possibly perform at a super high level.

- All four of these negative self-talk methods can cause an athlete to function well below ability levels. Worse yet, these patterns of behavior can become habits and affect all or most of an athlete's future performances, even until the end of their career.

- A person can significantly alter their beliefs and performance outcomes through mental training because the mind cannot distinguish between what is real and what is imagined if the imagination is vivid. This causes the brain to believe the scenario visualized has already happened and the athlete can grow immensely in confidence as a result of the brain believing it can and has been successful. This means that an athlete can alter and improve their confidence level. It also means athletes don't have to rely completely on outside successful experiences to shape their self-belief. Few athletes realize that confidence can be manufactured.

- Mental training mirrors physical training in that it takes time, consistent practice, and quality repetitions. It has to be viewed as every bit as important as the daily physical workouts are.

- Very few athletes partake in a regular, systematic protocol of mental training and ones that do can achieve a huge advantage over their competitors that do not. With dedication and work that advantage can be yours.

STEP TWO: ACKNOWLEDGE AND EMBRACE THE NEED FOR ENHANCED PSYCHOLOGICAL ABILITY

If we had to point to one factor that would enhance your athletic performance beyond any other, it would have to be sports psychology. Granted, performance is affected by many factors such as genetics, nutrition, off-mat preparation, psychomotor development, training, etc. However, if you were to ask any athlete (and we have done this with thousands of athletes from all over the world, for decades) what percentage of their sport is mental, you would hear that they believe a VERY large percentage is mental. The typical response is between 70-100%! We have never heard one say nutrition, sleep, vitamin supplement program or set and rep scheme in the weight room is 100% responsible for the outcome of an athlete on the field. Obviously, we cannot determine exactly what role any of these factors contributes to a definitive figure, but we fully agree that a significant part of success is derived from the mind/mental state of the athlete.

We must, therefore, take a closer look at psychology. The fact is, most athletes are not paying enough attention to psychological factors, nor do they know how to use psychology to enhance performance. Despite the fact that the majority of coaches and athletes that we mentored/coached feel that the psychological aspect of sport is extremely important, they more often than not ignore this in training. They talk a lot about psychology, but they rarely practice what they preach, as in, having a set routine like they do in physical skills practice. It is strange. Many of the world-class athletes' train three to six hours a day for as many as six days a week. They push themselves to their physical limits and then return the following day for more. When they are not training, they are either talking or reading about how to increase their performance. They spend hours watching YouTube and their competitors. They use any new age device they can find or afford that promises to increase performance. Nevertheless, during the 30 to 40 hours per week that these athletes are involved in their sport, usually not one hour is consciously spent preparing for the psychological aspects of the sport, as in: dedicated mental training on a logical, systematic progression to optimize mental performance. This does not make sense. Does it make sense to you, that a significant percentage of one's performance outcome is based off mental ability, yet there is no formal plan in place and dedicated training program to improve in that area? Thus, on the surface at least, there appears to be a great inconsistency between coaching philosophy and coaching practice. Obviously then, what makes psychology so important to an athlete is that it is a highly relevant and beneficial variable, but also a much-neglected variable.

Of course, this begs the question, "Why is such an important aspect of performance neglected by most athletes and coaches?" There are a number of reasons for this inconsistency, but perhaps the lack of knowledge concerning psychology is the most salient factor. The fundamental reason for this stems from a lack of formal training. Many coaches and athletes have taken only one introductory or no college courses in psychology and have not been exposed to this field as a science. Hence, most of the coaches and athletes' knowledge of psychology is based on personal experience and unscientific sources. Everyone knows to "train hard," "train harder," and "out-work your opponents," so this becomes the focal point of off mat training. Mass media sources emphasize the unusual and sensational fringe areas of psychology, which deal with topics such as behavioral problems, silly stage hypnosis tricks or therapy for mental illness. The few articles that do appear in sports publications or sites are often devoid of a useful, systematic approach to problem solving.

One reason for the lack of sound information is that most psychiatrists or clinical psychologists are not that knowledgeable about sports. Their educational training delves mainly into societal malfunction, and not performance optimization. Very few psychologists have ever participated in highly competitive athletics. They are not familiar with the obsessive pursuits, aspirations, or motivations typical of most athletes (nor are they concerned with such things). Their writing generally revolves around clinical patients who have deep-seated emotional problems. In short, they are more concerned with the abnormal than the normal. This is a far cry from those willing to risk life and limb to be extraordinary. In essence, their take on psychology is as far from an athlete's mind as the east is from the west. Consequently, such individuals do not know how it feels to make a comeback from a serious injury or what it is like to perform under extreme pressure. Nor do they know what it is like to fail or win at an important competition, or for that matter, what it's like to really exert oneself physically.

Psychologists may read about these experiences or observe them, but there is a big difference between those vicarious experiences and the real thing. In reality, they are worlds apart. In a nutshell, because of the aforementioned, most athletes and coaches perceive athletic performance as primarily a complex physiological process. Thus, coaches and athletes are more preoccupied with the physical and often ignore the mental and sociological. The problem with this viewpoint is that the athlete, like any human being, is a complex, unified and integrated living system. Therefore, behavior is a function of physical, mental, and sociological aspects. There is so much more than just putting another ten pounds on that bench press!

It stands to reason then, that we can only reach an optimum level of performance when we account for the physical, mental, and social factors that influence performance. That is to say we must perceive ourselves as an incredibly complex system which contains a body and a mind and which functions among and reacts to those who surround us. If we focus on only one aspect of performance, chances are that we will significantly limit our performance capabilities. Only when all systems are considered can we reach our optimum parameters.

So, one more time, just for emphasis...what makes psychology so important to coaches and athletes is that it is a highly relevant factor that is all too often neglected. Indeed, a very large part of your outcome will come from the mental component. Hopefully, you're motivated to continue on and learn how to bring about the next level.

ACTIVITIES

1. Write down all the things you are doing systematically and consistently to improve your mental game. ____

____

____

____

____

____

____

2. Interview three renowned coaches in your area to determine what systematic methods they are using to help their athletes mentally/psychologically. Summarize what you found. __________

____

____

____

____

____

____

____

3. Interview three renowned athletes in your area to determine what systematic methods they are using to help their performance mentally/psychologically. Summarize what you found. ____

____

____

____

____

____

____

____

4. Discuss your views concerning the importance of psychology in sports. ____________________

____

____

____

____

____

____

____

STEP 3: CREATING THAT VISION!

Over sixty years ago Dr. Maxwell Maltz wrote an incredible book called *Psycho-Cybernetics*. The major premise of the book was that the mind functions like a computer. The title of the book suggests that very concept. 'Psycho' refers to the mind and 'cybernetics' means computer...the mind is a computer. Within no time, the book became a bestseller. Perhaps you've read it. If not, you should. It's one of the most fascinating books you'll ever read. It was way ahead of its time.

Besides being an outstanding writer, Maltz was also a nationally renowned plastic surgeon. Actually, he was one of the best plastic surgeons in history. His work has been written about in all sorts of journals and there is even a number of training videos out that were produced by the medical profession so that other surgeons could study his work. The man was an absolute artist with a scalpel.

During his years as a surgeon, Maltz observed that individuals who had a congenital facial defect or those who suffered from an actual facial disfigurement as a result of an accident generally had a very low self-esteem. They were typically introverted, anti-social and extremely insecure. Their vision of themselves was horrible. In fact, many of the individuals whom Maltz interviewed refused to leave their home during the day, and when they did go out, they took great pains to hide their disfigurements. You don't have to be Sigmund Freud to figure out why these individuals acted that way. It's the Cooley's Looking Glass Principle. This principle states that we tend to make judgments about ourselves by looking through the eyes of others. Unfortunately, when most people come in contact with an individual who is atypical, their initial reaction is to turn away and/or try to avoid the individual. The individual with the deformity is taught that he is not acceptable. As Maltz observed, this feeling of non-acceptance is easily generalized to other psychological feelings such as worthlessness and inferiority. Maltz reasoned that since his subjects' deformities caused their poor self-images, by correcting those deformities, he could improve their self-images. Not surprisingly, Maltz decided to test his theory. There was no one better suited to make the physical improvements.

Dr. Maltz got together a number of individuals deemed "disfigured" and put them through a battery of psychological tests. As he had expected, the subjects' psychological profiles indicated that they had extremely poor self-images. He then went about correcting his subjects' disfigurements via plastic surgery. He literally re-sculpted their faces. When he got done with them, they were distinctly different, many having gone from the traditional "ugly duckling" to the "beautiful swan". Maltz was that good with a scalpel.

Unfortunately, things didn't work out exactly as Maltz expected. Although Maltz transformed his subjects from "ugly ducklings" into physically attractive individuals, they still perceived themselves as being ugly. They were drastically changed, improved, enhanced, but their vision was that their appearance and self-worth was still really poor. Maltz eventually realized that not only did he have to correct his subject's physical disfigurements with plastic surgery, he also had to correct the way they thought about themselves. He had to correct their VISION.

Now, here's the really good news. Once the subjects were taught to act and think positively, their personalities changed. They became more confident, outgoing, and assertive. And do you know what? They also started looking at themselves as being more attractive and appealing. In conclusion, it really never was about the physical abnormality. It was about each person's VISION.

There was another brilliant scientist named Victor E. Frankl. To say he was a scientist is an understatement. The fact is, he was a Medical Doctor and Psychiatrist, as in Victor Frankl, M.D., Ph.D. Think of him as a super genius. He was.

Unfortunately for Frankl, he was imprisoned in Nazi concentration camps, three of them. One of those was the worst of all, Auschwitz. During the time of these camps, it is estimated 5-6 million people died there, and typically about 6,000 died daily from starvation, beatings, disease, and downright acts of cruelty. It was among these prisoner beatings, starving and psychological abuses that Frankl kept a secret diary. He studied how some men lived, despite being merely skin and bones, while others perished. He wanted to figure out why some, who were not that particularly strong, fit or gifted, were able to survive, while others who seemed much more suited to survive, died. Remember, this was hell on earth, where prisoners ate bugs, and some even ate their own dead countrymen because it was the only "source of food" they would get.

Frankl's conclusions were later revealed as a Holocaust survivor in his book, *Man's Search for Meaning*. He concluded that the prisoners who had meaning and a sense of responsibility in their lives seemed to survive the camp better than others did. For instance, he found that married men survived the camp better than single men because they had something to look forward to beyond the camp walls (returning home to their beloved spouse). They had a VISION of reuniting with their loved ones. Most single men envisioned nothing beyond the walls. Once the prisoners found a why or some reason to live (a VISION), they then seemed capable of adjusting to the horrid conditions in which they had to live. The men who lacked VISION and lost hope, usually died quickly.

These two examples of two extreme circumstances point to vision. Those with a correct and great vision do significantly better than those who have a poor vision or no vision. Your outcome will be the same. Create a vision in all of your endeavors. Albert Einstein (another super genius) said, "Imagination is everything. It is a preview of life's coming attractions."

ACTIVITIES

1. Write down 5 VISIONS you have for your life.

    1.____

    2.____

    3.____

    4.____

    5.____

2. Write down 3 VISIONS you have for your year.

    1.____

    2.____

    3.____

3. Write down 3 VISIONS you have for your season.

    1.____

    2.____

    3.____

4. Write down all the available assets that you can use to achieve the VISIONS you selected.

____

____

____

____

____

____

____

____

____

____

STEP FOUR: PLANT SEEDS TO GROW INTO A MORE POWERFUL MIND

Now a few words about your mind…you know, that "sometimes amazing, sometimes a mess thing above your shoulders." It's in there alright and it is the most powerful weapon you have. It's been said that just about everything can be achieved through the mind -- health, wealth, happiness, and yes, even physical power. Without question your mind is an awesome instrument, far more powerful than your body. Once you learn to unleash the untapped reservoir of power in your mind, there is just no telling how great you can become. Not optimizing the ability of the mind is one of the greatest mistakes that an athlete can make. Selling the mind short, unfortunately, is exactly what a lot of athletes do.

Now, as you should be well aware of, your brain functions just like a computer. Well…that's kind of an understatement. Actually, your brain is a lot more sophisticated than any computer ever built. Do you know how many storage units are contained in that six-inch area on top of your shoulders? Ten billion! That's billion with a B. In order to construct a computer as comprehensive and sophisticated as your brain, it has been estimated by cybernetic experts that a company like would need a storage compartment as big as the Empire State Building to house it and enough electricity to light up New York City for a week to run it for an hour. It's mind-boggling (pun intended) when you think about it.

Here is something else you may find interesting. Some brain researchers estimated that even the most accomplished men of our time, guys like Albert Einstein, Michelangelo, Bill Gates, and Stephen Hawking use only a fraction of their brain's potential. "If man used the full potential of his brain," says Dr. Steven Burnhart, a leading neurophysiologist, "he would most likely cross the parameters of mortality. He would become God-like." Now that's certainly a thought to ponder.

If we accept the mind-computer analogy (and there is a prolific amount of neurophysiological research that indicates that we should accept it), then we must also accept the major premise governing the science of cybernetics. Briefly and simply, that premise states that computer performance is directly related to computer input. In other words, our brain and/or computer will respond directly to the way it has been programmed. If we fill our brain with positive, happy thoughts, we will respond in direct proportion to that programming. In essence, we will tend to be positive and happy. Conversely, if we bombard our brains with negative thoughts, we will respond negatively. It's the old garbage-in equals garbage-out principle.

Of course, if we respond directly to the way our brain has been programmed, it will only make sense that we would want to program our brains in a positive manner. The obvious question then is, "How do you program a human computer?" That's easy. It works the same way computers work. In case you didn't know, computer language is actually a complex series of electrical circuits. At the input terminal of a computer (the keyboard), words are typed into the device. The computer then converts the input into an electrical current and circulates it through its memory banks. The typed "input" now an electrical current, is then modified by the attitudes and responses that have been previously programmed into the computer. After the incoming information is processed, it is sent to the output terminal (screen) where it is once again converted into words and numbers.

Since your brain is just like a computer and it is programmed by words, thoughts, and actions, it should be our goal that every word, thought and action be a concise, positive affirmation. We cannot emphasize that point enough. The environment in which we function, the people with whom we interact and the thoughts that we entertain are all data constructs by which we are programmed. Therefore, we should operate in an environment that is stimulating and progressive; the people with whom we interact should be enthusiastic and positive; the words and thoughts we entertain should be powerful and positive. There is no way around it because computer (brain) performance is directly related to computer input. Program yourself to be positive and you'll be positive. Program yourself with negatives, and you'll be negative. It's just that simple. Words heard, or in self-talk matter!

The words we use have an impact on the way we think. Of course, when we hear words coming from our external environment they are also converted into thought. Obviously then, words are pretty important. If you're like most people though, you probably haven't given words much thought. The first thing you need to realize is that words have no meaning in their own right…they are simply symbols. We give words their essence and meaning. Consequently, the power and influence that words have on us are directly related to our social conditioning. Let us explain. If we say to you "stand up," most likely you would not envision in your mind's eye the letters S-T-A-N-D-U-P, but rather an image of yourself standing up. In short, the mind converts the words we use into mental images. The body then responds appropriately to what the mind conceives. It's the old axiom "what your mind conceives, your body believes".

This very concept has been consistently demonstrated in laboratory experiments that were designed to study the effects of autogenic training, a relaxation technique. Subjects who were told to visualize their limbs as being heavy consistently brought about heaviness in their muscles as measured by an electromyography. The reverse was found when the subjects were instructed to visualizing the sensation of lightness in their limbs.

Other studies have revealed that words and/or thoughts could raise and lower body temperature, secrete hormones, dilate, and constrict arteries and raise and lower pulse rate. Such research indicates the power that words can have upon performance and the need to be conscious of the language we use. Unfortunately, few individuals are aware that words can have a significant effect upon performance. Now you know. So, the first thing you need to do is to start using powerful positive words to build a powerful mind and body.

Muhammad Ali, one of the greatest strikers in history said, "if my mind can conceive it, and my heart can believe it, then I can achieve it." Simple statement, but it is very profound. Ali talked himself into success, whereas many athletes so often talk themselves out of success with self-talk like these examples: "That fighter is a world champion." "That gal destroyed me last time." "Look at the size of that guy." "This girl's kicks look so much faster than mine." We are programming failure by talking ourselves into a submissive role and putting our opponents into a position of dominance. Hence, we can either program ourselves into a superior or inferior position.

A great example can be found at the YouTube link: http://www.youtube.com/watch?v=FT-pfZAQvxw

It's Muhammad Ali's press conference from before his fight with George Foreman in Zaire, Africa. As a little background info for you: George had just fought the heavyweight champion, Joe Frazier, and knocked him down seven times! Everyone in the world knew Foreman was the biggest, baddest man on the planet at the time, and everyone felt he was unbeatable. The press conference is an amazing part of boxing history and a teachable moment for all athletes. For years when I watched this I saw "a cocky man belittling his opponent and making a jerk out of himself." That's what I believed I had seen until Dr. Judd Biasiotto, a Sports-Psychologist and record-setting powerlifter told me what was really happening psychologically. Both of us agree that a public forum was probably a bad choice for this discussion. It did indeed paint Ali as cocky and that is completely inappropriate for him or anyone else. Sadly, that's what people take away from this clip: him being cocky. What was really happening was Ali was doing something most athletes never do – he was talking himself into success. Athletes almost always talk themselves out of success, but Ali was talking himself into it. What a huge advantage. Re-watch it. Ali talked about beating a man who "hit harder than George, had a longer reach than George and was a better boxer than George," Right there are three positive affirmations. He mentioned he's a better fighter now, he's tough, professional, "bad" and that he has new training techniques, five more positive affirmations. He saw himself dominating alligators, whales, lightning, thunder, rocks, stones, and bricks. That's conquering seven impossibilities. Further, he's so mean, "he made medicine sick." No man has ever done that. Four times he said how fast he was and told himself he was faster than the response of a light switch. Finally, he called himself GREAT. Did you count twenty-two instances of Ali programming himself for dominance? Dr. Judd did. Perhaps that's why Dr. Judd used Ali's technique called "psychic driving" enroute to him squatting more weight than any drug-free powerlifter in history at forty-four years of age: he squatted 603 pounds at a bodyweight of only 130 pounds! Again, it wasn't the cockiness. It was a bad forum to sound cocky. What it really was, was brilliance. He used psychic driving to program his subconscious mind for a superhuman performance, which is exactly what happened when he knocked out Foreman. Use discretion but use psychic driving too. Talk yourself into superhuman results. As English heart surgeon Martyn Lloyd-Jones stated, "Most of the unhappiness in life is due to the fact that you are listening to yourself and not talking to yourself."

Obviously, there is a big difference between having hopes of being great and actually believing that you are going to be great. Once you believe that you can be great, achieving your goals is just a short step away. Belief is the magic elixir that can transform mediocre individuals into world-class human beings. Believing opens the doors for success. Anyone can do amazing things regardless of who they are or what their circumstances are. They can become or do almost anything they want if they put their minds to it.

As the saying goes, "If you think you can, or you think you can't, you're right." There is magic in believing. You are what you think you are, and you become what you think you will become. We don't want to belabor this point, but it's just that simple. If you believe, you can go beyond what other people think is your breaking point; you most likely will transcend that barrier. In fact, you can go beyond even what you may think is your breaking point...if you believe. Let's say it one more time...you can do almost anything if you put your mind to it. If you believe, there is just no telling what heights you can reach.

Of course, the question is "How do you get to the point where you really believe in yourself?" The answer is so simple that we are afraid to tell you for fear that you will stop reading. You see most people are looking for complex answers to simple problems. They tend to let their minds get in the way of their progress. Consequently, when you give them simple solutions to their problems, they tend to dismiss the answer because it sounds too simple for it to work. Worse yet, they look at you like you're crazy. With the hope that you will see things differently, we are going to tell you the secret to believing in yourself. Think positively! That's right, think positively.

As mentioned, the mind is a highly sophisticated computer with awesome potential, but just like computers, it's only as good as its programming. If you program your brain with negative affirmations, you're going to respond negatively (garbage in equals garbage out). However, if you program your mind with positive affirmations, you're going to respond positively. It's that simple. Like we already mentioned, you are the sum product of the events you experience...the environment in which you function, the people with whom you interact and the thoughts that you entertain, are all data constructs by which you are programmed. If you constantly entertain positive thoughts and events, you will develop a positive mentality. There is no way around it.

The great thing is that positive thinking always works if it's used properly. The problem is that many times people don't understand the nature or process of positive thinking. Positive thinkers do not deny that negative things happen or that failure exists. They simply refuse to dwell on such events. Rather, they look for the positive element in each situation and build upon it. Concisely, positive thinking is a form of thought, which habitually siphons the positive element in each situation and builds upon it. Note also that seeking the positive is a deliberate, systematic process. It takes effort and concentration. It requires hard work, perseverance, and discipline. It is not easy to perfect, but positive thinking will work if you are willing to work at it.

A word of warning concerning positive thinking...it's not magic. There's no way you're going to break a state, national or world record just by thinking about it, especially for a very brief period of time. Sitting around thinking that you're great won't make you great. Let's face it; there are indeed guys sitting around in mental institutions who think they are God! Those guys aren't exactly setting the world on fire. Belief is ineffective without action. All of the positive thinking in the world won't make you great, but positive thinking, sound goals and hard work over a deliberately scheduled mental training protocol work will. You can believe that.

You can use psychic driving every day. When you wake up each morning, tell yourself that you feel strong, powerful, and happy. Also, tell yourself that you can do anything. Then constantly reinforce these concepts throughout the day, always suggesting that you are great and that there is nothing you cannot do.

Eventually you will believe it! In order to get the most out of psychic driving, there are a few suggestions you might want to follow. Research has revealed that the most effective affirmations are ones that are both believable and vivid. Experimental studies have also found that spontaneous suggestions, those that capture the true feelings of a successful experience, are the best to utilize. Consequently, power words such as "I feel strong and powerful...I feel confident and self-assured" are good phrases to use right before you have to perform in a pressure situation.

Words like "easy," "relax," and "calm" are important when trying to maintain your composure before contests.

Be careful of negative self-talk. As mentioned, research has consistently revealed that negative talk will produce undesirable effects upon an individual's self-concept and performance. Unfortunately, most people are not even aware that they make negative statements, nor are they aware of the powerful impact that words have on their feelings and behavior. For this reason, it is imperative that you are aware of the dialogue you use. In fact, the key to enhance control of self-talk is to become aware of what you say to yourself. If by chance you find yourself saying something negative, stop yourself, analyze why you used a negative and manipulate it into a positive affirmation. By self-monitoring your words, you will eventually be able to eliminate the negative and focus on the positive.

A modification of psychic driving is a method called scripting. Scripting is a written and/or recorded dialogue, which is designed to enhance self-confidence and performance. You can write and re-write the same script every day, or you can record onto your phone and play the script several times daily. It's a good idea to write your own scripts. Be careful to say words and statements that will elicit the emotional response you want at that particular time. Get the hang of making statements that elicit totally positive images. Here is one psychic driving script a national champion wrestler we coached would use: "I am fast. I am powerful. I deserve to be the national champion and I can beat anyone because I train longer and harder than anyone in this country. I set up all of my attacks with blinding speed and confidence. No one finishes attacks better than I do." Note how this is one hundred percent in a positive affirmation. Everything is positive.

Avoid all negative words in scripting, such as "don't," "not," "no," and so on. For example, "I am not tired" would be better phrased "I feel fresh and energetic." Using words like "tired" can trigger mental images of being tired and flood the subconscious with bad images. Remember, it is the job of the subconscious to merely act out on what is programmed into it. It is critical to flood it with positive images. Think of words that motivate or emotionally stimulate you. These words are known as "trigger" words. One way to find trigger words and positive statements is to review books on positive thinking.

Many individuals who use scripting to enhance their performance listen to their recorded scripts prior to their training sessions, or prior to competition, in order to get mentally prepared for what they have to accomplish. As mentioned, the more you use positive affirmations, the more positive and powerful you will become. It is a good idea to have different scripts available and use them randomly.

"Reach high. Vision big. Achieve big. You are capable."

ACTIVITIES

1. Go on a seven-day diet of positive thinking. For the next seven days make an honest effort to bombard your mind with positive affirmations. When you wake up in the morning, think that you are strong, powerful, and happy whether you feel that way or not. Throughout the day, reinforce these feelings and thoughts. If at times negative concepts enter into your mind, stop yourself from dwelling on those thoughts, analyze why you are having them, and then manipulate them into positive affirmations. Also, in a small notebook write down all of the negative words and thoughts you are entertaining during this time so that you become more aware of the negatives you are using. ____

____

____

____

____

____

2. Develop a list of trigger words that are extremely motivational to you. _______________

____

____

____

____

____

____

3. Write two different motivational scripts that you can use to enhance self-confidence and performance. ____

____

____

____

____

____

____

____

____

____

4. Record the aforementioned scripts so that you can listen to the tape prior to your workouts, prior to competition and during your mental training sessions.

STEP 5: DEFINING YOUR GOALS

Hopefully you now have some visions that inspire you. Think of these as your "grand hope" for your journey. This is the place every journey should begin. Hopefully now you also understand the need for a superior mental game and the infinite power of the mind. Now we're on to the serious stuff: goals. Goals are not visions. Visions are ideas or actions that may drive us towards a happier or more fulfilling future, for example," I want to take a vacation." It's an idea.

Goals on the other hand are definitive destinations. Think of them as your road map to get to your vision...or should we say phone app map since times have changed? The goals might be, "I really want to go to Atlanta" (broad goal). If I take I-10 east for seven hours I will get to El Paso, TX., where I will have lunch. Then I will fill up my tank and get back onto I-10, etc. These are smaller goals that lead to the bigger goal (getting to Atlanta), that helps fulfill the grander vision (taking a vacation). Goals defined, according to Wikipedia, are "desired results that a person or a system envisions, plans and commits to achieve: a personal or organizational desired endpoint in some sort of assumed development."

Going back to one of our super genius, Victor Frankl, we can take a closer look at goalsetting. Frankl knew about the superiority of those with vision, those who committed to setting goals. After Frankl was released from the Nazi concentration camps, he devised a therapy, which he called "Logotherapy". Basically, Logotherapy is a goal-oriented therapy, which is based upon the premise that in order to be successful in life, an individual has to have meaning and direction in life. Frankl believed that people who had no real goals in life had little meaning in life and without meaning in life, they had no life. Only when an individual had purpose and direction in life would he be in a position to succeed, to really live. Interestingly, Frankl's theory has been consistently validated by research studies conducted in America. In fact, there is a wealth of research, which indicates that the most successful and happiest people are those who are goal oriented. Generally, people who have a definite purpose or goals tend to be most successful.

Of course, goals are not just visions. They are visions that are formally planned out and acted upon. Goals are the seeds to success. If you have no idea where you are going in life, how can you expect to get there? Goals give you a way to get to your destination. The road to success starts with setting goals to achieve the grander vision.

Before we go on, we are going to give you a few quick suggestions to help you to set your goals in the future. First of all, set goals that are both realistic and flexible. Don't set a goal that is so impossibly high that you ensure failure. Athletes do this all the time. In fact, research studies have shown athletes to fall short of their goals as often as ninety percent of the time, and that's not because they aren't training hard. It's because they set their goals too far out of reach. Goals should definitely stretch you. If you aren't put on edge, there is no real accomplishment. Vision big. Think big. Set big goals but set realistic goals!

On the other hand, goals cannot be made that are too easy to accomplish. Goals that are too easily accomplished are not ideal for making huge performance gains. Achievement of worthy goals also takes time, so you will need to be both patient and persistent. Many small steps taken consistently add up to a significant amount of success. This was proven unequivocally by

James Clear in his book *Atomic Habits*. It Is a book every athlete, and every person for that matter, should read.

Once you establish your goals, write them down and check them off as you accomplish them. This will not only serve as reminder of your daily routine, but it will also shape your actions by reinforcing these small bits of behavior. Often the achievement of your goals will include a number of other considerations.

On the sheet listing your goals, outline obstacles that you may encounter while trying to achieve your goal. These obstacles may include physical weaknesses, time constraints, coaching or knowledge you must obtain, or accessibility to other resources. For instance, increasing your explosiveness and speed for karate may require that you develop a systematic program of auxiliary strength exercises designed to enhance overall power production, speed, and rate of power production. Some of your goals might entail nutritional planning to ensure weight gain or weight loss, increasing the biomechanical efficiency of your kicking, or implementing the various types of strength training routines you might need to follow. Once again, be realistic. If you are competing as a novice, do not expect to be a World Champion next year. All sports require a lot of time and energy to be successful. Do not get discouraged. Remember, it is not what you start with in life that counts, but rather what you end up with. With a goal-oriented program, and prolonged, serious work, there is no reason why you cannot realize your true potential.

After you have identified the obstacles to each goal, identify the people who can help you achieve your goals. This list may include family, coaches, training partners or subject-matter experts such as psychologists, nutritionists, researchers, or technical advisers. Along these same lines, save room for yet another column that identifies training aids, supplements, and other outside essentials for performance optimization.

Once you have charted this information, you can now construct a game plan that will help you to deal with obstacles effectively. The idea is to devise a systematic approach to reach your goals in the most efficient way. With this type of game plan in hand, all that's now required is action on your part. That's the hard part. Merely writing a goal down does not guarantee that you will achieve it. You have to go out there and get your hands a little dirty if you are going to be successful. Whatever you do, don't expect immediate results, and don't get discouraged. Champions are not built in a day. Chances are you won't be either. Be patient and persistent. Develop the habits it takes to improve daily. Remember that in education, business, and sports, as in life, it's not what you start with, but rather what you end up with that is important. Start out slow, be systematic, work hard and before you know it, into the stars you go. Let nothing stop you! Mission accomplished! Goal fulfillment!

ACTIVITIES

1. Write down 5 long range goals that you would like to accomplish this year.

    1.____

    2.____

    3.____

    4.____

    5.____

2. Select one of the aforementioned goals and develop primary and secondary goals that you would use in achieving that goal.

    a) Primary Goals: ____

    b) Secondary Goals: _______________________________________

    c) Long Range Goals: ______________________________________

3. Write down all the obstacles that you may encounter in your attempt to accomplish the goals you selected. ____

4. Write down all the available assets that you can use to achieve the goals you selected. _____

5. Using your primary and secondary goals, along with your obstacles and assets, write out a specific game plan to reach your goals. ______________________________

STEP SIX: MASTERING RELAXATION TO CALM THE MIND AND ENHANCE VISUALIZATIONS

If you're human, you're going to experience anxiety and stress during some time in your life…it's something that comes with the territory. Anxiety can range from mild forms of apprehension to paralyzing terror. How well an individual handles anxiety and stress is many times the difference between poor athletic performance and peak performance. It is widely accepted that if an individual's anxiety level is too high, the individual will be unable to attain an optimal level of performance. Obviously then, it is imperative that we learn to control our anxiety levels.

Psychologists have experimented with various techniques to control anxiety and stress. Deep muscle relaxation was one of the first methods used. Basically, it was used as an incompatible behavior to reduce anxiety. The rationale behind the use of deep muscle relaxation as an incompatible behavior is that relaxation and anxiety are antagonistic to each other. In other words, it is impossible to be relaxed and stressed at the same time. Consequently, whenever you experience anxiety at an inappropriate time (like pre-match), you can reduce or alleviate that emotion if you induce deep muscle relaxation.

The rationale behind using deep muscle relaxation to desensitize stress and anxiety is rather ingenious. When an individual achieves deep muscle relaxation, he cannot experience anxiety and/ or the physiological arousal associated with the stimulus. Thus, by continually pairing an anxiety or fear-provoking stimulus with deep muscle relaxation, you can eventually learn to relax in the presence of that stressful stimulus.

Of course, the aim of deep muscle relaxation is not for you to become totally devoid of the stresses in your environment. The purpose, rather, is for you to feel comfortable with yourself and alert to your internal and external environment. The idea is not to put you in a total stupor, but in a controlled physiological state. There are a number of methods that you can use. Here are a few that are the most convenient forms of relaxation that you should experiment with.

Plan A: Learning the Progressive Relaxation Technique

According to many psychophysiologists, this technique is one of the best manual relaxation methods that can be taught. The procedure requires neither special equipment nor a trained administrator and it can be performed in a variety of settings. Best yet, it is easily learned.

First, find a nice quiet room where you will be free from the distractions of television, telephones, people, gremlins, and most importantly, social media for at least an hour (yes, this is humanly possible). Having selected your practice room and time, lie flat on your back with your arms at your side. Next, close your eyes and as an aid to concentration, keeping your eyes closed for the entire session. In this technique, you will practice direct muscle relaxation by learning to recognize when tension and stress are present in various muscle groups. Then, you will learn how to bring about deep relaxation of these muscle groups by engaging in a series of exercises.

The first thing you are going to do is learn to recognize the sensation of delicate muscular contraction. After a few minutes of quiet rest, direct your attention to your right hand and very slowly begin to bend your hand back at the wrist. As you do this, concentrate on the way the back of your hand feels. You want to detect the first slight indications that something is happening…

this feeling is "slight tension". If you feel sensations in the upper arm or biceps, you are making too much of an effort. If that is the case, put your hand back on the bed, rest a few minutes, and repeat the procedure. Be sure that the sensation you feel is in the back of your hand and not the front. Note also, always rest between trials so that fatigue is not a determining factor in your performance.

Once again, remember that what you want to detect is the first slight sensations of tension that you experience when you bend your hand back. The objective is for you to learn to recognize this feeling whenever and wherever it occurs in your body. This is not as easy as it might sound because tension signals are very slight, fleeting, and they can be difficult to recognize at first. Don't rush through the procedure. Take your time, and make sure that you identify the sensations of tension before you go on. Note, several practice sessions may be necessary to master this sensation for some individuals, and that is perfectly fine. Do this with your fingers, toes, quadriceps, and all of your muscles, achieving "slight tension," in many different body areas.

When you are positive that you can identify the sensation of tension no matter where it should occur in your body, you are ready to learn to recognize the next higher level of sensation… the sensation of strain. Once again, you will have to lie down on your back with your eyes closed and your arms at your sides. After a few minutes of quiet rest, lift your right arm so that your forearm is vertical while your elbow rests on the surface of the bed. Slowly bend your wrist back towards your shoulder. As you do so, concentrate on the sensations in your forearm. Do you recognize these sensations? We hope so because it is tension again. If you did not, please re-read the previous three paragraphs. Now, direct your attention to the back of your wrist. Pull your wrist back very hard towards your shoulder as far as it will go and hold it there. Make the muscles that are contracting as tight as you can. You should be experiencing a new feeling, a new sensation distinctly different from tension. This is "strain". Strain is like tension on steroids. It is a sensation where you contract the muscles hard and cannot hold for very long.

The sensations of slight tension and strain only vaguely resemble one another. You should have little difficulty distinguishing between them. You'll need to repeatedly observe these sensations until you have distinctly recorded them in your memory banks. If you persist, if you work hard and diligently, you will be able to detect these sensations in a mere fraction of the time that it took you during the early stages of observation and experimentation.

Having recognized the undesirable (strain), you must now reverse the process of creating tension and strain and arrive at the absence of muscular tension…a state of relaxation. The important thing to realize about relaxation is that no effort is required to reach this particular state. That is the secret…no work, no effort! As if your source of power has failed and your muscular structure has disintegrated, the feeling that you are ultimately seeking is a complete lack of tension and strain.

Once again, assume a reclined position with your arms at your sides and your eyes closed. You ought to have this down by now. After a few moments of quiet rest, direct your attention to your right hand once more. Just as before, slowly bend your hand back at the wrist. Immediately, you should be able to detect the slight sensation of tension. Don't stop though. Bend your hand back as strongly and far as you can. The sensation you are experiencing now is, of course, strain. Hold your hand in this position for about ten seconds, and then, "turn off" your source of power. To do so, you must relax instantly and completely.

To better illustrate what it would feel like to "turn off" as you have been instructed, picture yourself exerting all your strength in an effort to push a large boulder off a sheer cliff. When suddenly, the boulder goes over the edge, there is no active resistance to your pushing and all your straining instantly ceases. It is that feeling of nothingness after the boulder drops that you are striving to obtain when you "turn off" your source of power. Once you have done so, let your arm drift back to your side and concentrate on this feeling of relaxation. Remember, you want achieve nothingness, no worries, no effort...just complete physical relaxation. Relax a few minutes and try once more. Do this same exercise over and over until your mind can evoke the feeling of deep relaxation. Practice recalling this sensation until you are positive that you can recognize it and produce it without going through the actual exercise.

Now it is time for you to put it all together. Your awareness of tension, strain, and relaxation are all part of the effort to produce total body relaxation. The first thing you will need to do is to find a quiet and comfortable room where you will be free from intrusion or phone calls for at least an hour. A more conducive atmosphere for this type of experimentation is one that is dimly lit or even completely dark. Your body should be clothed in attire that is comfortable. When you are ready, lie down on your back with your arms at your sides and your eyes closed. A pillow or rolled up towel could be placed under your neck and under your knees if desired. When you tighten the muscles of your body, try to think of these muscles as being made of rubber, rope, or rubber bands stretched tightly. Also, try to adopt the attitude that when you relax your muscles, your body will continue into deep relaxation, even after you can no longer feel it do so. After a few minutes of quiet rest, direct your attention to your toes because this is where we are going to start. Curl your toes under and squeeze them very tightly. Do you remember that sensation? You better, it's strain.

While you hold your toes in that position, try to visualize the muscles that you are using. Think of them as if they were rubber bands being stretched tightly across your feet. Now, ever so slowly and passively, let them relax. Visualize these muscles going limp as if being drained of all their strength. You are seeking that sensation of relaxation, that feeling of nothingness.

Next, extend your toes and bring them towards your body. Tighten up these muscles so that you are aware of the areas and the sensations involved...remain very tight and very tense. And then let them go... "power off."

Your legs are next. Push them straight out with your heels towards the floor and your toes pointing straight ahead. Tighten up your calf and thigh muscles as if they are rubber bands pulling tight. Concentrate deeply on the sensation there and let them go...total relaxation, limp, calm, light, and tranquil.

Now, concentrate on your gluteal muscles. Push your lower thighs against the pillow that you placed under your legs, tightening up all the muscles of your buttocks. Make these muscles very tight and very tense as you concentrate on the sensations that you are experiencing in these muscles. After holding this position for a period of time, slowly and progressively relax the muscles. Remember the feeling of relaxation...the zero feeling. Take a deep breath and hold it. At the same time, arch your back slowly, tightening the muscles of your back. Concentrate on these muscles, thinking of them as if they were strong rubber bands pulling tighter. Focus your attention on the sensations that are taking place within them.

Next, slowly exhale loosening up the muscles of your back. As you do so, think, "power off." By this time, you should know the feeling you wish to experience.

Your arms are next. Lift them gently off the bed, fingers extended. tightening the muscles in your arms, slowly make a fist and squeeze your fingers together very tightly. Visualize the muscles pulling tighter and tighter. Now, ever so slowly, begin to bend your elbow, bringing your fist towards your shoulder while keeping the muscles in your hands and arms very tight. Keep thinking of these muscles as being stretched tight. At the same time, be cognizant of the sensations that you are experiencing in them. Slowly and passively let your arms drift back to your sides, turning everything off, nothingness...the zero feeling.

Now move your head forward until your chin touches your chest, tightening up the muscles in the back of your neck. These muscles are very close to the nerve trunks descending from your brain. Therefore, they are of particular importance in relaxation. Concentrate on the muscles you are using and the sensations of tension that exist. Once again, slowly, and progressively relax these muscles, letting your head fall back to a comfortable position on the bed.

After accomplishing the above, squeeze your forehead muscles tightly. Think of the muscles you are using and the sensations that are involved. Relax and let your muscles drift into the "zero state."

Work next on the speech region. Put your lips together as if you were blowing up a balloon, tightening your facial muscles as you do so. Feel the muscles pulling tighter. Concentrate on the sensations that are involved. Hold this position momentarily and blow out the air, letting your muscles go limp and loose, feeling total relaxation once again.

Finally, tighten up all the muscles of your body at once. Point your toes straight in front of you and push your arms straight into the air. Arch your back slightly. Put your chin on your chest and blow out your cheeks. Gradually, contract all of these muscles, visualizing them growing tighter and tighter. Concentrate on the sensations in these areas and completely turn yourself off. Let your feet go limp, let your arms drift lazily back to your sides, your head back into the pillow, and exhale. Just let yourself sink into nothingness, the "zero state", complete physiological relaxation.

This should bring about a very deep feeling of relaxation--one much deeper than normal. Remember, this skill will develop more and more with time and repeated practice, just like your sports skills did. Once again, patience is the key. Don't rush it! An encouraging note is that once you have learned the skill of deep muscle relaxation, it is yours for the rest of your life.

Plan B... Learning Meditation

Another method that can be used to induce deep muscle relaxation is meditation. First of all, you need to plan a program just as you would for effective physical development. One or two sessions a day, one in the morning and one in the evening is what many people who meditate use. Begin with 5-10 minutes for one session daily and gradually work up to 20 minutes for one or two daily sessions. Some individuals have found that meditating right before going to work or physical exertion gives them a boost. Others say that meditating right before going to bed is best for them. This will be something that you will probably have to decide on your own. The important thing is that your meditation sessions should be regular, and you should not miss any of them. Don't meditate right after a meal. Sit in a comfortable position and be in a place where you won't be disturbed.

Assume a comfortable sitting posture in which the head, chest, and shoulders are held erect and straight. Your posture should be comfortable so your body can remain still throughout the duration of the exercise. Once you are comfortable, begin to pay attention to your breathing. Count slowly as you inhale, "1, 2, 3, 4." Now, count slowly as you exhale, "1, 2, 3, 4." Each number you count should take one second. You will find that your inhalation lasts about the same number of seconds as your exhalation. The normal ratio of inhaling to exhaling is 1:1. It should take you about 4 to 6 seconds each way. Now, let's change that ratio to 1:2. Inhale for 4 seconds and exhale for 8 seconds. Concentrate and count the seconds. The reason for making the exhalation twice as long as the inhalation is so you can get maximum control of your lungs. Therefore, squeeze out all the carbon dioxide gas and waste products that are in your lungs. No matter how hard you inhale, unless all the carbon dioxide is squeezed out of the lungs, you cannot bring in a significant amount of oxygen. In ordinary breathing, we squeeze out only a small portion of air from the lungs.

As you meditate on breathing, be aware of how you breathe. You should be "belly breathing", where your abdomen expands and contracts, and not "chest breathing", where your rib cage moves up and down vertically. Use your whole respiratory system, leaving no portion of the lungs unfilled with fresh air. The inhalation process should begin with the downward movement of the diaphragm into the abdomen. Next, the abdomen is expanded, and the upper part of the lungs is inflated as the rib cage is expanded.

If you're breathing correctly and are able to achieve the 1:2 ratio of inhalation to exhalation, you are ready for breath retention. Inhale for 4 seconds, hold your breath for 4 seconds and exhale for 4-8 seconds. You can gradually increase the seconds as you gain more competency. The inhalation-retention-exhalation of one breath is called a round. Perform 15 to 20 rounds during each session. If you are able to do this easily, you have excellent control over your lungs and your power of concentration is superb! End each meditation session by sitting quietly for a few moments, breathing normally, and experiencing the effects of this type of meditation. After meditation, most people feel not only relaxed, but step in breath meditation...alternate nostril breathing.

Plan C: Developing Your "Relaxation Ring"

One of the tips you can use is to create an associated reflex by forming a relaxation ring. This is a great tool to have in your "emotional toolbox" for times when you feel contest or pre-contest nervousness, and you don't have a quiet room to retreat to.

To create the ring, you will have to practice learning how to relax several times. You now know how to do that. Once you become more proficient, put yourself into an environment where you would normally practice the progressive relaxation techniques. Start the relaxation process. Your goal will be to create a relaxation ring, using your hand, ten times and each time achieve a total body relaxation state one level deeper. It goes like this: lie down and, lay with your palms up and gently curl your ring finger to your thumb. Do this slowly, gently, freely, without tightening up. When the ring finger gently touches the thumb, exhale slowly and feel yourself going into a deeper state of relaxation with less muscle tightness throughout your entire body. Allow the hand to slowly drift open. While staying relaxed, repeat the procedure nine more times. What you are really doing is pairing a signal to relax with the ring hand configuration. Done enough times, this will cause an automatic calming and sense of relaxation when you need the technique and need it due to stress, like before games, during games, when you get super winded, etc. It is an amazing little tool athletes don't know about that can prevent you from making huge withdrawals in your emotional piggy bank due to nervousness.

So how does all of this help me?

First, the deep muscle relaxation induces a hypnotic-like state in which the brain frequency cycles per second are greatly diminished. It is when these cycles are greatly slowed, and the mind and body become relaxed that the brain can go from a Beta state (14-40 cps) to an Alpha one (7-14 cps). This is a great way to reduce your stress and interestingly enough is a more advantageous state for the visualizing we are going to talk about in order to optimize our mental training. The more relaxed you are, the better you can visualize. The better you visualize, the more success your brain perceives. The more success you perceive, the more confidence you will have. The more confidence you have, the bigger advantage you will have over your opponents.

Second, the ability to learn to relax is critical to control the pre-contest jitters that all athletes get. Every athlete gets only so much emotional energy that is stored in an emotional type of piggy bank. Those that use up lots of energy in worry are continually making small withdrawals from that bank. When the heat of competition later on gets tough, there simply are no reserves left. Those who can remain calm pre-game have greater stores of energy left for the championship minutes of their contest: the very end.

1. Explain the significance of using relaxation techniques to enhance athletic performance. ___

____

____

____

____

____

____

____

2. Practice the aforementioned two relaxation methods in depth and determine the pros and cons that are specific to your needs. _______________________________

____

____

____

____

____

____

____

____

STEP SEVEN: PROGRAMMING YOUR COMPUTER: VISUALIZATION PRACTICE

Quite a few decades ago Dr. Brian Fisher and a few of his colleagues at Michigan State University were sitting in the lab when all of a sudden Brian got this interesting idea. His idea was to investigate what went on in the brain when it was having an experience. The people in the lab got a number of subjects together and hooked them up to an electroencephalograph (EEG) so that they could record their brain waves. While the subjects sat in the lab all wired up, the experimenter introduced them to various experiences: a pretty woman, a gunshot, a woman's scream, and a dog running across the room. After each experience, they checked the reading on the EEG to see how the brain responded. After a number of trials, one of the researchers got another idea. He theorized that the brain responded to physical events in the same manner that it responded to conceptualized events. For instance, when the subject watched the dog walk across the room, light from the dog was converted to electricity at the subject's retina, passed over his optic nerve and then, stimulated his brain. Consequently, the subject saw the dog. The dog was envisioned in the subject's brain even though a dog outside his body caused it.

The question next posed by the researchers was, "How would the brain respond if the subject just visualized the dog walking across the room?" They decided to find out. The subjects were then blindfolded and asked to visualize the dog, the pretty woman, the gunshot, and the woman screaming. When the brain waves recorded for the imagined experience were compared with the brain waves recorded for the real experience, they found them to be nearly identical. What did this mean? Simply put, the brain and/or nervous system cannot distinguish between an experience that is real and one that is imagined, if the imagery is done well. It only follows then, that an imaginary experience is just as much a conditioner of attitudes, habits, and responses as a real experience. Consequently, if an individual closes his eyes and vividly visualizes himself performing a particular behavior, his brain will actually process that information in the exact same manner that it would if he had performed that behavior in real life.

That's not all. It gets better! A researcher at the University of Texas named Sherman Smith later discovered that not only will mental imagery (picturing) condition our mind, as mentioned, but it will also condition our body. What Smith found was that when the brain conceives of an idea, it generates impulses throughout the body, which facilitates neurons of the body to perform the idea being conceived. For example, Smith showed that when weightlifters lie down and visualized themselves performing a lift, the imagery actually resulted in subliminal activity in the muscles associated with the imagined performance. The muscles were contracting as if they were actually performing the lifts.

To illustrate this concept further, let's assume that as you visualized yourself performing a roundhouse kick (of course, any skill could be visualized), there was someone in the room observing you. As he watched you run through this mental conceptualization, he would see no muscle movement in your shoulders or arm. However, if he hooked your hip flexors, glutes, and quadriceps to an electromyography (EMG), he would not only be able to get a muscular reading, but he would actually be able to tell which muscle groups were coming into play during the conceptualized version of the kick. Of course, the strength of the impulse is not as strong as one that is being generated through actual performance, but that is inconsequential.

The fact is neuromuscular activity is present. The beauty of this is that by visualizing your performance, you are actually doing two things that will make the real "skill" easier. First, since the brain cannot distinguish between what is real and what is imaginary, you are programming your brain to believe that you have actually executed the behavior, thereby increasing your self-confidence… assuming that what you visualized was that of a positive nature. Second, you are also programming your body because as your brain conceives of performing the behavior, there is a cortical spill over (brain messages) which facilitates the neurons in the body to perform the idea that is being conceived.

Perhaps best of all, because there is no physical taxing of the body, a fighter can throw hundreds of kicks and punches in visualization, programming success, without overtraining the body.

Guidelines for Visualization Training

In order to use mental imagery (visualization) effectively, there are a few simple guidelines you will need to follow:

1. **Induce Deep Muscle Relaxation.** Research has consistently revealed that imagery combined with relaxation is significantly more effective than imagery alone. Actually, relaxation is an excellent method for desensitizing fear and anxiety. Remember that relaxation and anxiety are antagonistic to each other. It is impossible to be anxious and relaxed at the same time. When an individual achieves deep muscle relaxation, she cannot experience anxiety and/or the physiological arousal associated with the stimulus. Thus, by continually pairing an anxiety or fear-provoking stimulus with deep muscle relaxation, the subject will eventually learn to relax in the presence of the stressful stimulus. We have already detailed the need for deep muscle relaxation prior to visualizing and will talk more about the significance of relaxation in the chapter on stress management. Still, it is an important concept to understand, and sometimes saying things more than once drives the point home. Know that even if the situation is not that super stressful, it is still to your advantage to mentally rehearse your performance while under deep muscle relaxation because, in essence, you are developing an association reflex between your performance and deep muscle relaxation. In this manner, your chances of being calm and composed while engaging in the behavior will be greatly enhanced. The ability to bring about deep muscle relaxation while in stressful situations will not only improve your performance in those situations, but also allow you to resist burning up valuable energy by controlling your anxiety level.

2. **Visualize as vividly as possible.** Research has revealed that the more vivid an individual can visualize the behavior he is practicing, the more significant the improvement. As mentioned, individuals differ in their ability to form mental images. Some individuals can visualize in high definition and color, others in black and white and some individuals claim that they can only think in words rather than in pictures. As with any skill, the ability to visualize will improve with practice. The more you practice, the better you will get at producing vivid imagery. When you visualize something, you should be able to focus on the image vividly. You should be able to see the image, its shape, color, texture, imperfections, variations and all the sensations associated with it. In imagery training, the visual, auditory, olfactory, taste,

tactile and kinesthetic senses are all important. By using all your senses, you will be able to create more vivid images. Even the emotions associated with your various experiences are important in practicing imagery. In using imagery to desensitize anxiety, fear or anger, you must be able to recreate those emotions in your mind. One thing that you can do to improve your visualization skills is to become more observant. Tips are listed below in the chapter activities for how you can improve this skill. When you are training or competing, take mental notes of your surroundings. Try to become more aware of all the sensations that are present… sights, sounds and smells. Also, try to be more conscious of the feelings you are experiencing during this time. Focus on your strengths: feelings of power, confidence and success are the types of feelings you want to mentally record. It's a good idea to mentally rehearse successful experiences right after they occur, if possible. Close your eyes and vividly see the skill that you have just performed. Once again, make sure that your mental images are as you would see them through your own eyes. It cannot be overemphasized that, as with any skill, the more you practice, the more proficient you will become. In brief, the more you visualize, the more your visualization skills will improve.

3. **Be realistic about what you visualize.** For instance, if you are typing 20 words a minute, you wouldn't want to visualize yourself typing 150 words a minute. Research has revealed that unrealistic imagery is significantly less effective than imagery that is realistic and consistent with the individual's ability. Obviously, mental imagery is not magic. It will not take you beyond your genetic parameters. In a word, it is better to visualize a performance that is just out of reach rather than imagining one that is completely unrealistic.

4. **Never use imagery that is negative.** Visualize only positive mental images. Remember that you can learn negative responses as well as positive ones. Consequently, never picture yourself doing inappropriate mechanical skills. Always see yourself as being confident, relaxed, and positive. We cannot over emphasize that, as with any skill, the more you practice visualizing, the more proficient you will become. In short, the more you visualize, the more your power of visualization will improve. With a little imagination, you can see how this type of conditioning could be used to increase your self-confidence, motivation, and assertiveness. Better yet, it grants you the ability to program your mind and body to act as a positive person would act. Think, act and most importantly, see yourself as being confident and self-assured.

ACTIVITIES

Activity 1

As indicated, visualization is one of the most important aspects of your training. This first exercise was basically designed for someone who has never used visualization or has very little experience with the technique. That does not mean it is going to be easy to master or that it is insignificant. Actually, it may be the most important activity in this section. The first thing you want to do is deeply study something very familiar to you like a red apple. An apple is a very easy object to focus on but understand that you can use any object that you are comfortable with. Study it from all angles. Recognize the color, its skin, and its imperfections. Recognize that "red" apples aren't exclusively red. Next, induce deep muscle relaxation. Once you are deeply relaxed, visualize the red apple. Recognize the color, its skin, and its imperfections. Recognize that "red" apples aren't exclusively red. They have many hues. Don't let distractive thoughts get in the way of visualizing the apple as clearly as possible. Visualize the apple from all angles possible, point to point. Notice how your red apple is red, green, yellow, brown, gray, white and even black in some small places. It is not simply "red." Once you can visualize the apple clearly, without distractions, we are ready to move on. Do not move on until you can see the apple clearly without any distractions. It may take you a number of sessions before you get to that point. Don't get discouraged. It takes practice. Once you are able to maintain a clear image of the apple without any distraction, we are ready to move on. Open your eyes and cut the apple down the middle. Observe the particulars of the apple in great detail. What's its color? Count the seeds in its core. Observe the contrast of the black seeds with the soft whitish-yellow color of the apple's inside. Smell the apple and notice any other specific details about your apple.. Once you have mastered all these details vividly in your mind's eye, we are ready to complete our first step in our visualization training. Open your eyes, sit up and taste the apple. Concentrate vividly on the taste of the apple, how you are chewing it and even the saliva in your mouth. If need be, take a couple bites. Once you feel that you have all the specifics in your mind, lie back down, close your eyes, induce relaxation, and then visualize everything we previously talked about. Understand that perfecting this exercise may take numerous sessions. Whatever you do, don't move on until you master this activity.

Activity 2

As mentioned, when you are training or competing, take mental notes of your surroundings. Try to become more aware of all the sensations that are present...sights, sounds, and smells. Also, try to be more conscious of the feelings you are experiencing during this time. Each night lie down, induce deep muscle relaxation and visualize your training sessions for the next day. See everything as vividly as possible: your biomechanics, sights, sounds, and smells. Spend at least 20 to 30 minutes on your training session. The more time you engage in training the better. You know the old saying "practice makes perfect"? It is false. Practice makes permanent. Only perfect practice makes perfect. You want your visualization training to be perfect. Don't wing it, perfect it. This is a hard task, but well worth the many hours of practice you will put in. When aforementioned Sports Psychologist/Powerlifter Dr. Judd Biasiotto was trying to beat the best lifts made in the world as a drug-free powerlifter, he would use visualization each day without fail to prepare himself for both his practice sessions and his competitions. His story is incredible and perfectly illustrates the power of the mind and visualization. For instance, each day before practice, he would induce deep muscle relaxation and then visualize himself going through his entire workout for that day. Judd would conceptualize everything as vividly as possible...the gym, the weights, even his coach. He actually perfected his visualization skill to the point that he could smell the odors associated with the gym. Other competitive lifters we have coached have reported the same sensation after deliberate practice. During his mental sessions, Dr. Judd omitted nothing: he visualized himself warming up, stretching, loading the bar, and making every rep of every set. He would rehearse his workout routine in this manner many times during each session. Sounds like a lot, but get this, from his own words, "Believe it or not, when I was training to break the 600-pound barrier in the squat, I would mentally rehearse my performance over 500 times during each week of my mental training sessions. By the time I attempted the record, I estimated that I had rehearsed that lift over 30,000 times," he further declared. It is no wonder why he squatted 603 pounds, weighing only 130 pounds. He had been there 30,000 times before and had 30,000 successes. His brain was flooded with success. His brain knew without doubt he could make that lift. Of course, that number seems exceptionally high, but keep in mind that the visualization of a performance is much quicker than the physical performance itself. In essence, you can program your body through visualization at a much greater rate than you can through the actual physical performance of the lift.

Activity 3

As previously mentioned, the ideal way to visualize is internal visualization, where you picture your performance through your own eyes as if you were actually performing it. It was also mentioned that an individual's ability to visualize is subject to variation. Some see in high-def color, others in black and white. Both are ok. For some, external visualization is much clearer and becomes a preferred method. Note, while scientists who study this for a living recommend internal visualization as a preferred method, they also report that external visualization can be just as effective for some people. If this is your case, know you can still make huge gains in your mental programming. Here's how: visualize, or if you will project, an astral being coming out of your body. The astral being would be in your very image; as in, it is you! See him/her very distinctly. It is as if he is real and not just a part of your imagination. Watch your conceptualized double perform your desired skill with picture-perfect form. Replay the scenario hundreds of times, as this engrains picture perfect technique and also the confidence that you have done it and will do it. Focus on your strengths: feelings of power, confidence, and success are the types of feelings you want to mentally record. It's also a good idea to mentally rehearse successful experiences right after they occur, if possible. Try this external visualization every night for a week and take delight in how much your skill improves in this area.

STEP EIGHT: REDUCING YOUR STRESS

All athletes suffer from stress, and karateka are no exception. Stress is inevitable. Being stress-free is not a worthy objective because it is not attainable. The issue isn't how to eliminate stress because you can't. The issue is how to make it manageable and non-performance changing. How do we best respond to anxiety provoking stimuli?

It is believed that by pairing relaxation with an anxiety provoking stimulus, the subject will eventually learn to relax in the presence of the stimulus. South African Psychiatrist Joseph Wolpe, a foremost authority on behavior therapy, devised a technique to do just this. The good news is that the technique, which is referred to as systematic desensitization, has been widely used and researched over many decades. As a result, it has a very large research base. The majority of this research indicates that systematic desensitization is a very effective method for alleviating anxiety. Wolpe's program has three components: anxiety hierarchy construction, relaxation training, and scene presentation.

You have already learned about relaxation training. The next steps are to understand hierarchy construction and how to appropriately present the anxiety provoking stimuli for optimal results in desensitization. Anxiety hierarchy is creating a list of anxiety-producing events which have been arranged in an array from least to most anxiety-producing. For example, suppose you experience extreme anxiety in the morning of tournament day. Every time you experience anxiety in relation to that tournament, you would immediately record the circumstances surrounding the anxiety-provoking situation. You record what you think caused the anxiety, where you are, what you were doing, who you were with, and the situation at hand. The more information you have concerning the anxiety-provoking situation, the better. Once you identify an anxiety provoking stimulus, rate the stimuli on a scale of one to ten with one being the least anxiety provoking and ten being the most anxiety provoking. After recording such stimuli for a period of two or three weeks, you would construct your hierarchy.

For example, below is a modified hierarchy constructed by a National Champion female karateka who complained of anxiety associated with fighting during competition.

1. The nervousness of making weight all week before a tournament.
2. Losing sleep the night before the tournament, worrying if all of the needed gear is packed.
3. The energy rush when arriving at the tournament site.
4. Walking through the doors of the competition site and seeing the other fighters.
5. Warming up for the event and thinking it won't go off on time.
6. Being called to the ring for the first round.
7. The entire first fight.

This hierarchy was condensed from a list of dozens of potential anxiety-producing stimuli. Of interest is the fact that fear of not packing all of the needed gear was more stressful to the fighter than the fights afterwards. This is more common than you might expect. In fact, most individuals reveal that the anticipation of an event is usually more stressful than carrying out the event. In other words, the actual participation is less anxiety-provoking than thinking about participating.

Here's how to proceed to gain control of these anxiety-provokers.

1. **Relaxation Training** is the first step in controlling anxiety (after the hierarchy construction) Achieve deep muscle relaxation. Of course, you know how to do this by now. Hopefully you have practiced this so you can achieve a fast deepening and very relaxed state, ideal for imagery.

2. **In-Vitro Conditioning** After you have become proficient at achieving deep muscle relaxation and after your anxiety hierarchy has been constructed, induce as deep a state of relaxation as possible. When you are totally relaxed, you will visualize the scenes on your hierarchy. This is called "in-vitro" conditioning. To start, visualize the scene that makes you the least anxious on your hierarchy. Visualize this scene for approximately 15 seconds. If at any time you get nervous or anxious while visualizing the scene, immediately terminate it. If termination of the stimulus is required, re-induce deep muscle relaxation, and repeat the visualization of the same scene. Continue this procedure until you can remain totally relaxed while visualizing the anxiety-producing stimulus. Once this has been mastered, move on to the next scene in your hierarchy and repeat the above-mentioned procedure. Continue in this way until all the scenes on your hierarchy have been desensitized. Note again that the anxiety-producing stimuli are repeated until you can visualize them without experiencing anxiety. Again, the rationale for the effectiveness of this procedure is that by repeatedly pairing anxiety-producing events with deep muscle relaxation, the visualized scenes become counter-conditioned or desensitized. Because of stimulus generalization, counter-conditioned imagined scenes correspond to behavioral improvement in the "real life" or "in-vivo" situation. In a few words, once you are able to relax while vividly visualizing yourself in an anxiety provoking situation, there is an excellent possibility that you will remain relaxed in the real-life situation.

   An advanced consideration is to then perform this entire procedure (deep muscle relaxation and in-vitro conditioning) in an environment similar to one in which you might compete, and feel is a stressor. For example, a karateka can do hours and hours on relaxation and in-vitro conditioning in a quiet, isolated room. Once this is mastered, they may wish to consider practicing both techniques at a dojo that is pretty serene. This brings them closer to the stress of the real competition but is a systematic progression from the sterility of clinical environment. A more advanced step is to perform the relaxation and visualization techniques in a chaotic situation like a tournament venue, even if you are not competing in that tournament.

3. **In-Vivo Conditioning**. Once you are able to visualize all of the anxiety producing stimuli on your hierarchy while remaining totally relaxed, you are ready for the real thing…in-vivo conditioning. Actually, the same procedure is used except that instead of visualizing the anxiety provoking stimuli, you actually engage in the activity that is causing the anxiety response. When you are totally relaxed physically, engage in the behavior on your hierarchy that makes you least anxious. Note that you should perform this behavior in the actual environment setting that is indicated on your hierarchy. As with your in-vitro or visualization conditioning, if at any time you become nervous or anxious while performing the behavior, immediately stop what you are doing and again induce deep muscle relaxation. Repeat this procedure until you are able to perform the behavior for three successive repetitions without experiencing anxiety. Once this has been accomplished, move on to the next scene on your hierarchy and repeat

the above-mentioned procedure. Continue in this manner until all of the scenes on your hierarchy have been desensitized. As noted, many times in-vivo conditioning is not necessary. Again, it depends on the specific situation and how well the individual responds to in-vitro conditioning. More often than not, once you are able to relax while visualizing yourself in an anxiety provoking situation, there is an excellent possibility that you will remain relaxed in the real-life situation. If that happens to be the case, in-vivo conditioning would not be necessary...you would be good to go. Stress: all competitors get it, and so do many of the referees.

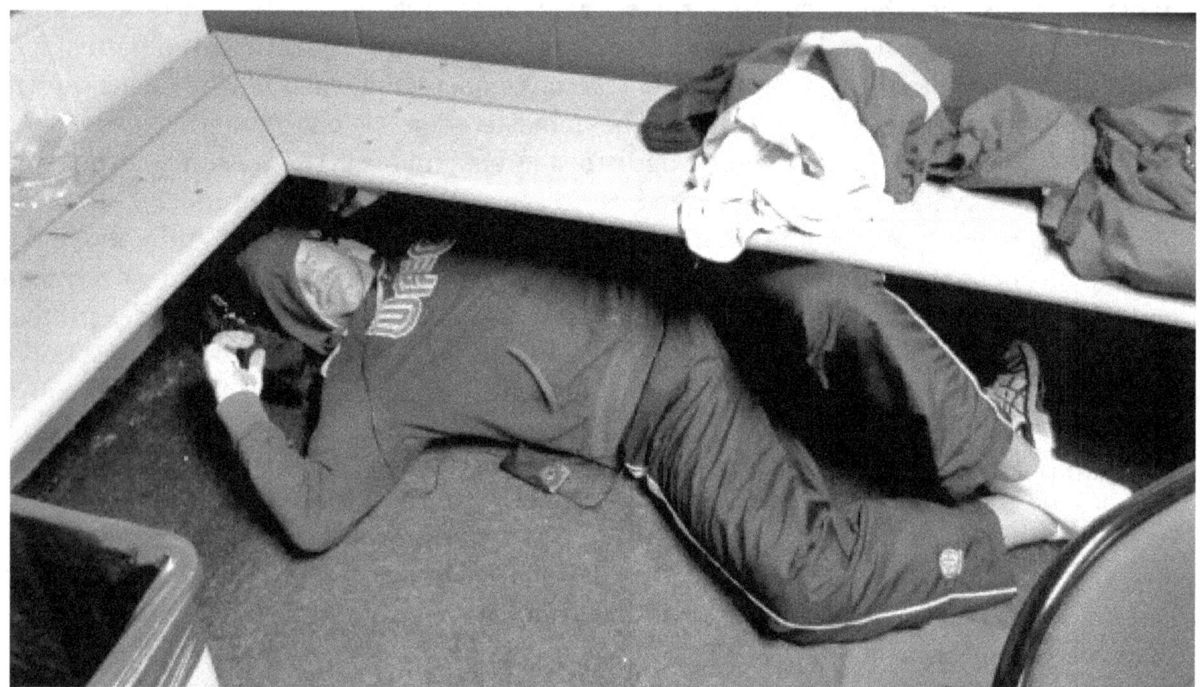
A great way to get away from the stress of fighting in the Ultimate Fighting Championships

ACTIVITIES

1. Explain the significance of using relaxation techniques to enhance athletic performance.
____
____
____
____
____
____
____

2. While everyone has stress, some people are more stressed than others and it is helpful to recognize your stressful areas so that you can do something about them. Below list typical areas of stress: ____
____
____
____
____
____
____

3. List people that can help you with stress related areas: clergy, sports psychologists, counselors, coaches and so on. _______________________________________
____
____
____
____
____
____

4. Construct an anxiety hierarchy for a specific activity that is adversely affecting you. _________
____
____
____
____
____
____

5. Using deep muscle relaxation, in-vitro and in-vivo conditioning desensitize the anxiety hierarchy you constructed above. _____________________________________
____
____
____
____
____
____

STEP NINE: GETTING INTENTIONAL ABOUT THE BENEFITS OF SLEEP

Getting a good night sleep is just as important as getting a good training session. Contemporary research has consistently revealed that sleep is an essential ingredient for a healthy and productive life. Even more revealing is that research indicates that sleep is one of the most important aspects in developing fitness and strength. It has been proven to be far more critical than anyone previously thought.

One thing remains clear, whatever sleep is, it is extremely important...especially to athletes! According to researchers Frederick Baekeland and Ernest Hartmann, the average person sleeps approximately seven and a half hours per day. Approximately five percent of the population sleeps less than six hours a day and another five percent sleeps more than nine hours a day if given the chance. Baekeland and Hartmann have identified these individuals as short sleepers and long sleepers, respectively.

From a physical standpoint, the researchers found that short sleepers sleep an average of 330 minutes per night. Long sleepers get about 527 minutes of sleep per night. Both groups averaged approximately 75 minutes of deep sleep per night, but long sleepers averaged almost twice as much REM sleep as did short sleepers. Why long sleepers need more REM sleep than do short sleepers is unknown. Baekeland and Hartmann believe that personality differences that were discovered between the two groups may be responsible for the different sleep patterns.

Since everyone dreams nightly, it can be assumed that dreaming serves some necessary function. It has been hypothesized that individuals who are under a lot of stress, or who are exposed to new and challenging situations, tend to need more dream time. Again, perhaps, athletes experience more stress than average individuals. Of course, this is only speculation, but physical training is a source of stress. So is the thought/reality of getting punched and/or kicked repeatedly.

Although no one knows what the function of sleep really is, it is believed that if an individual is deprived of REM sleep, the individual will experience ill effects. William C. Dement, a Stanford University scientist, proved that very point in a fascinating study that he conducted way back in 1960. Dement had his subjects sleep in his laboratory every night for a period of ten days.

While the subjects slept, Dement monitored their sleep cycles with an EEG machine. When the subjects were in a light or deep sleep, Dement did not disturb them. However, as soon as the subjects entered into the REM period, he would wake them up. After he woke them up from REM sleep, he would tell them to go back to sleep. In almost all cases, as the subjects went back to sleep, their sleep cycle started over again. They would go through light sleep, deep sleep and to REM sleep, at which time Dement would wake them up again. He continued this process throughout the night. Thus, his subjects got all the light and deep sleep that they wanted, but they were deprived of REM sleep and consequently, dreaming. After depriving the subjects of REM sleep and dreaming for several nights, they became more cranky, annoyed, impulsive, and hostile at times.

Dement also reported that the subjects experienced difficulty in learning new tasks and significant decrements in performance of already learned tasks. Interestingly, most of the subjects after a few days of REM deprivation, exhibited shortened sleep cycles. It was as if the subject's body was trying to rush through the light and deep sleep to get to the REM period of sleep. Dement speculated that the body was attempting to catch up on the REM sleep and/ or dreaming that it had been deprived of. Also of interest, was the fact that many of the subjects reported experiencing anxiety and nightmares for several nights after the REM deprivation was discontinued. Apparently, the loss of REM sleep triggered the nightmares. Furthermore, research has shown that it can take a month or more to repay the REM sleep debt that accumulated in a week's time.

As indicated, sleep deprivation not only affects mental preparedness, but also physical performance. There are several studies which have revealed that as little as two hours of sleep deprivation nightly for a period of one week can cause significant decrements in strength, speed, and coordination. Physiologists also believe that rest is just as essential to muscle growth as nutrition and proper exercise. Most athletes can usually control their diet and exercise routine. On the other hand, sleep is a factor which may be a troublesome aspect of their training regimen. Many athletes, even world-class athletes, often find it nearly impossible to sleep the night before an important competition.

Interestingly, there are several types of sleep disturbances. The most common disturbance is known as insomnia, or the inability to fall asleep within 20 minutes after going to bed. In one study, more than 30 percent of the athletes surveyed reported experiencing insomnia during some portion of their career. This is unhealthy for several reasons. It can cause lower energy levels during waking hours, reduce thought process ability, decrease coordination and a significantly reduce ability of the immune system to fight off illnesses. Further, it causes a decrease in testosterone production in some who don't get enough sleep, a factor that will greatly reduce power and recovery. None of these are beneficial to performance.

Unlike the previous chapter activities that have a sequence, all of these activities in this chapter can be done immediately.

Activity 1: Eliminate or reduce such stimulants as caffeine (coffee, tea, and soft drinks) and alcohol (wine, beer, and liquor) from your diet, or reduce the amount of them that you consume, especially after noon time. It goes without saying that if you take stimulants during the day, they might make you crash during the day or keep you awake at night. Although alcohol is a depressant and might induce drowsiness, it will interfere with your sleep cycle.

Activity 2: Create a good environment for sleeping. For instance, keep your room dark, have a good room temperature (65 to 70 degrees) and a comfortable bed. You can use aroma therapy and soothing music therapy if you choose, but nothing that pumps you up. It is a good idea to make your environment free from distracting noises such as television, telephone, and electronic devices. Next, turn off your phone; the Twitter, Instagram, Tik Tok and Snapchat addictions can be fulfilled in the morning.

Activity 3: Try to eliminate all the discriminative stimuli from your environment. Don't watch TV, eat, or read while in bed. In fact, you're best to get away from all electronics (especially those that light up, like phones, televisions, and tablets) an hour before you go to bed. Make sleeping a pure experience. If you have your TV in your bedroom, take it out this very instant!

Activity 4: If you are not sleepy, don't go to bed and don't stay in your bedroom. If you don't fall asleep in 20 minutes or so when you go to bed, don't stay in bed. Get up and go into another room until you are tired. In fact, try to stay out of your bedroom until it is time to go to bed.

Activity 5: Try to get into a relaxed bedroom routine before you sleep, hopefully void of electronics. Find activities that will calm you down and will take your mind off things that might excite you. You might also want to try relaxation techniques like progressive relaxation, meditation, and yoga to bring about a relaxation response.

Activity 6: Develop a sequence of activities into a pre-sleep ritual before going to bed. This is called "chaining". What you want to do is the same routine every night before going to bed like taking a warm shower, drinking a warm glass of milk (milk contains tryptophan, a natural sedative), putting on your Spider-Man jammies, etc.

Activity 7: Let go of things that happened during the day or what is going to happen the next day. Earlier in the day, write down all the things you want to do the following day so that this will not interfere with your sleeping ritual.

Activity 8: Try to go to bed every night and get up every day at the same time. Don't sleep in, even if you don't have to get up in the morning or if you slept poorly. If you do this, you probably will feel tired the next day, but it will be easier for you to sleep the next night.

Activity 9: Don't worry about falling asleep. There is what is called "the law of reverse effect" which states that the harder you try to do something, the more frustrated you will become.

You have probably heard the old cliché, "Birds of a feather flock together," or "You are who you associate with." Research has consistently shown that the people we surround ourselves with significantly influence our behavior. If we surround ourselves with positive and successful people, we will tend to be positive and successful. Conversely, if we surround ourselves with negative and ineffectual people, we will tend to be more negative and ineffectual. All of our actions, feelings, behavior...even our abilities, are consistent with our conditioning and/or socialization. We are the sum product of the events we experience...the environment in which we function, the people with whom we interact, and the thoughts which we entertain, are all data constructs by which we are programmed. Therefore, the environment in which we function should be stimulating and progressive. The words and thoughts we entertain should be forceful and positive. Program yourself to be positive and, you'll be positive. Program yourself with negatives and you'll be negative. It's just that simple. We tend to "act like" the type of person we are socialized to be. Not only that, but we literally cannot act otherwise, unless we make a conscious effort to do so. Obviously then, the way you are socialized will go a long way in determining how successful you'll be in athletics, as well as in life.

If you've been conditioned to believe you can, there's an excellent chance that you will. Conversely, if you've been conditioned to believe you can't, you most likely won't. In order to win, you must expect to win.

Here is a good example of what we are talking about. There was an extraordinary study called "Pygmalion in the Classroom" that was done a number of years ago at Harvard University. You can read about it in Leo Buscaglia's book *Living, Loving, and Learning*. A study was conducted to determine the effect that expectation had upon performance. These professors from Harvard went to a number of high schools and told the teachers that they had a test that could measure which kids in their class were going to grow intellectually during the coming year. The test was called the Harvard Test of Intellectual Spurts. The professors told the teachers that the test was the most valid instrument ever constructed to measure intellectual growth. "It will pick the intellectually gifted students right out," they said. "It never fails." So, the professors went into the schools and gave the kids some antiquated intelligence test. After the kids took the test, the professors threw them into the garbage. Then, they randomly selected five names from the teacher's roll book.

They took the names to the teachers and said, "These are the kids who are going to really excel this quarter. These are your gifted students." And the teachers looked at the list and must have thought, "This can't be. This kid here on the list exhibits no potential for high academic performance, and these over here just don't care. There is no way this group is going to be successful. You must be mistaken." The Harvard professors said, "Trust us. The test never fails. These are the kids who are going to progress intellectually during the year. You'll see." And the teachers looked at each other and thought, "These guys are from Harvard, they must know what they are talking about."

Do you know what happened? Every kid on the list grew beyond expectation. They went right off the charts, which just goes to show you that you get exactly what you expect. If you teach a child and you tell him he's dumb, you are going to get a child who lives down to your expectations, just as if you teach a child and tell him that he's smart or gifted, that child will live up to your expectations. The same is true of athletes. If you condition and teach an athlete to believe that he's a loser, you are going to get an athlete who lives down to your expectations just as if you teach an athlete that he's gifted, that athlete will live up to your expectations.

Here is something else that will interest you. Joe Burson did a number of great studies on reinforcement and how it affects performance. He would go to schools and videotape teachers while they were teaching in the classroom. It was a candid camera type thing where the teachers were unaware that they were being filmed. Burson would take the films home and study them carefully. What he found was amazing. Fifty four percent of the responses that teachers made to their students were negative. Isn't that sad? But listen to this, he did the same study with coaches, and do you know what he found? Eighty three percent of the responses that coaches made to their athletes were negative.

According to Burson, the coaches tended to ignore good plays by their athletes and consistently criticized poor plays. Haven't these guys ever heard that you can catch more flies with honey than you can with vinegar? Why concentrate on the negative all the time? Why not build everyone up instead of dragging him or her down? Get rid of the vinegar and use a little honey. On second thought, put a lot of honey in there.

What does this tell us? Simple, it tells us that we are a product of the people we surround ourselves with. Consequently, it is imperative that we surround ourselves with positive people, in a positive environment. If anything, society influences an athlete's behavior.

This may sound very harsh but if the situation you find yourself in is not allowing you to reach a level of excellence and self-fulfillment, then it most likely is time to get to know people who are in alignment with your dreams. We are not suggesting that you abandon your friends, but rather to surround yourself in training with people who have similar goals and aspirations... people who appreciate the things that you want to accomplish. The right people can elevate you to a higher level...inspire you to achieve your goals. You want to find people who can really share in the journey, people who will hold you accountable, and people you can hold accountable. Surround yourself with positive people. Surround yourself with success!

ACTIVITIES

1. Write down your goals and desires. Start by making a list of the traits or characteristics that you really desire. Determine if the athletes you are surrounded by have the same ambitions and aspirations that you have. ____

____

____

____

____

____

____

____

2. Ask yourself, is my circle of influence empowering me to become the person I want to be? ____

____

____

____

3. Critically ask yourself: am I in a situation where I can get the most out of myself? __________

____

____

____

4. Critically ask yourself: do the athletes I train with inspire me and challenge me to be better? __

____

____

____

5. Consider your past and present. List the people you surround yourself with, are the relationships reciprocal? Is there a healthy give and take in your relationship with these people? __________

____

____

____

____

____

____

____

____

____

6. Name your limits for negativity among your immediate group. You can't set good boundaries if you're unsure of where you stand. So, identify your physical, emotional, mental, and spiritual limits. Consider what you can tolerate and accept and what makes you feel uncomfortable or stressed. Those feelings help us identify what our limits are. ________________________

____

____

____

____

____

____

____

____

7. Look at the people in your surroundings (not just athletes) that you're spending time with the conversation that you're having and if it's helping you to create the career you want. This is not always an easy thing to do because we're creatures of habit and we're comfortable in relationships that are familiar to us. Are these people helping you make the decisions you want to make, learn the things you want to learn, become the athlete you want to become because if they aren't then you may need to consider how much time you spend with them. You don't need to cut them out completely, but you may need to assess the time you have and the value you're getting from that relationship. One true test is to think about how you feel after you've spent time with them. Do you feel energized, excited about your decisions and on the right track or do you feel drained and depressed? ____

____

____

____

____

____

____

____

STEP ELEVEN: STRIVE FOR PERFECTION, BUT LET GO OF IMPERFECTIONS

Perfection. What an incredible ideal. Think of having the perfect body, the perfect match, the perfect tournament. Wouldn't life be great?

Forget about it. You cannot have it. The fact is you cannot have any of those things. Perfection does not exist. And yet, so many athletes are obsessed with it. Why are we so obsessed with an utter impossibility?

The ideal of perfection is...well... a perfect ideal. We should all strive for perfection; in everything we do. The pursuit of perfection and unwillingness to accept anything less can be a competitive edge that separates you from all other competitors. From that standpoint, the ideal of perfection is proper.

Where it goes off course is athletes beating themselves up after imperfect performances. This is the sin. Remember, you cannot have a perfect performance. It does not exist. When you hold yourself to that standard you are certain to fall short. In falling short, one typically becomes self-critical. The brain acts out upon this garbage you are programming into it—that you always fall short. This is when performance suffers and guess what.... you start the cycle all over again by trying to be perfect next time. You are essentially circling in the proverbial toilet bowl, on your way down.

Rather than focusing on perfection of technique, athletes should focus on perfection of effort. This can be controlled. This is a worthy goal. This is the path that can best optimize your performance. Granted, this is hard, super-hard, crazy-hard. To continually give your very best is a painful, different path. But this path is attainable. This is in your control. The greatest conquest of all is of oneself, as Plato said.

Note: Previous all-time home run champion and Hall of Fame legend Babe Ruth actually struck out more than anyone in the history of baseball.

NBA legend Michael Jordan, considered by many to be the best basketball player in history said, "I've missed more than 9000 shots in my career. I've lost almost 300 games. 26 times, I've been trusted to take the game winning shot and missed. I've failed over and over and over again in my life. And that is why I succeed." In fact, this is a staggering statistic: of the top 15 players in NBA history, 10 are in the Basketball Hall of Fame. The other five aren't eligible because they haven't been retired long enough to be eligible... but they're all going to be in it. The list of those in the Hall that made the list of most career missed shots includes Kobe Bryant, LeBron James, Michael Jordan, Wilt Chamberlin, and Kareem Abdul Jabbar. Fourteen of the fifteen players on the most missed shots list were named by *The Atlantic Magazine* on their list of the top 75 players in history.

The point is you have to have a long memory and a short memory simultaneously. It's important to have a long memory to remember the successes and how they came about, so that you can replicate the process. It's important to have a short memory to not engrain the mistakes. Those are better off not dwelled upon.

The only worthy goal is you bringing out your very best, first as a person, and second, as an athlete. Never forget the words of some of the finest minds in history:

"Nothing can stop the man with the right mental attitude from achieving his goal; nothing on earth can help the man with the wrong mental attitude." -- Thomas Jefferson

"Human beings are made so that whenever anything fires the soul, impossibilities vanish. A fire in the heart lifts everything in your life." -- John C. Maxwell

"Every great and commanding movement in the annals of the world is the triumph of enthusiasm. Nothing great was ever achieved without it." -- Ralph Waldo Emerson

"Until intelligent thought is linked with appropriate action and follow through there is no real accomplishment". -- Brian Tracy

"Never let the odds keep you from doing what you know in your heart you were meant to do." -- H. Jackson Brown Jr.

"Have great hopes and dare to go all out for them. Have great dreams and dare to live them. Have tremendous expectations and believe in them." -- Norman Vincent Peale

MENTAL PROGRAMMING SUMMARY

By now you should have a pretty clear understanding of how to proceed with a mental training program that can give you a HUGE advantage over your competitors. Never forget, the essence of sports is to separate individuals. You have to be separated. You are guaranteed to be separated. You win or you lose. It's that simple.

You are the Chief Executive Officer of your present and eventual outcomes. While you may not be able to do anything on earth you wish to do, like out-run Usain Bolt, the fact is you can be almost anything you truly want to be, anything in which you fully dedicate your heart and work with full intention to achieve. To pursue a purpose without pause is the true secret to success… one aim, without halt, no excuses, no apologies, no quitting, just total unremitting resolve in achieving your objective. It is the quality of commitment that separates the good from the great… little else. When you are committed to excellence, when you have an attitude that screams out "NOTHING LESS THAN THE BEST," then you are on the road to greatness.

Every journey is merely an opportunity. They are all opportunities to strengthen you, to help you evolve, to create a better person and athlete. Since the most worthy goal is to bring out our best, we should all step up any time an opportunity presents itself. The first step is to create an awesome vision, one that stretches us, one that puts us on edge to attain, but will bring peace of mind and heart once the work is done and the vision is fulfilled.

 We know this will take immense work. Hard work is not the way we get there. Everyone works hard. If we merely do what they do, we will likely have the same outcome. Rather, we need to put in unrequired work, going above and beyond what others do. Without extra effort we cannot have extra joy. "Until intelligent thought is linked with appropriate action and follow through there is no real accomplishment."

Once the vision is set, we need definitive goals. Goals are merely wishes until they are carefully and deliberately written down. When short-term and long-term goal planning is complete, we prepare the complete athlete, physically and mentally strong. One without the other is sure to help us achieve only part of our potential. To bring out our very best we need to put forth our very best effort in trying to optimize both mental and physical systems. We need superior relaxation skills, visualizing ability and a positive environment. We need to value sleep and time off. We need to give our best effort in eating better than our opponents.

The mental system is not currently being optimized in most karateka. If you choose to do so it would give you a huge competitive advantage over those who are not. Remember, the brain essentially acts like a computer. It is programmed by thoughts, words, and perceptions of past experiences. The law of computers says it will spit out whatever is programmed into it, good or bad. It is therefore critical for your total development to flood your mind with positive affirmations and beliefs: stronger than any your opponents may have. Your goal is to beat them, to go above and beyond what they do in this area of development. You have to first beat them at this task to later on beat them in the arena.

This program will take time. You didn't become great at karate overnight. It has taken you years or decades of hard work to increase your proficiency. We should never forget the gallons of sweat, the heart breaks, the frustrations, broken bones, and agony. You're going to need to apply the same heart and effort to your mental training—this is part of the deal. Also never forget, you get out what you put in. The more you put in, the more you put out.

Only one gets to be called champion. Be that one. The choice is yours.

A Model for
Lifetime Progression

7

Karate & Sport for Life is a philosophical approach for age-appropriate training. *Karate & Sport for Life* can be integrated into anytraditional based Karate-Do curriculum. Istvan Bayli and Richard Way developed the foundation of this program in their highly successful LTAD (Long Term Athletic Development Program), which is being used across the sports spectrum in the UK and a number of other countries.

Following the successful hosting of the 2002 Olympic Winter Games, the Utah Athletic Foundation (UAF) was formed to nurture a legacy of Olympic winter sports in Utah. This effort produced the Utah Sport for Life Program. Utah Sport for Life will employ a collective community-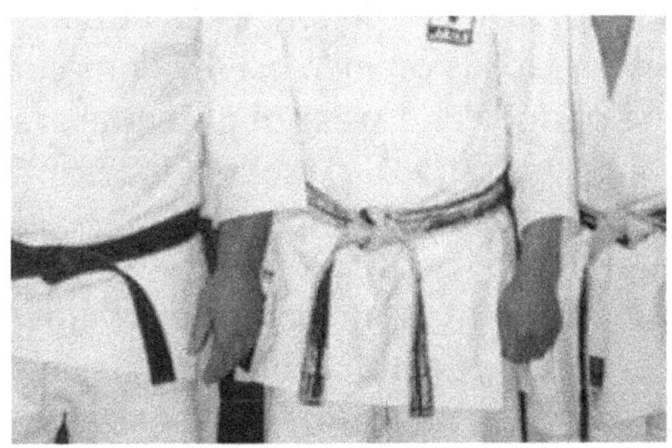wide effort to elevate Utah's quality of life through participation in sport and recreation. Jepperson Karate Dojos and Park City Karate were invited to teach at the Sports FUNdamental Camp 2009. From this experience and numerous seminars with Dr. Istvan Bayli, we have developed the *Karate & Sport for Life* program. This outline is an effort to identify some critical windows of development during every child's life. The goal is to integrate science and traditional karate-do for the benefit of the student.

Parents and martial arts instructors are in a unique position to help young people learn the principles of success in life and athletics. The "DO" arts in Japanese martial arts, emphasize mental strength and discipline. Before any successful athletic career can happen, mental discipline must be developed. In fact, success in any endeavor in life is predicated on the discipline and persistence.

Many authors have published books on the components of success and expertise. *Outliers*, by Malcom Gladwell, *Talent Code* by Geoff Colvin and *Nurture Shock* by Po Bronson & Ashley Merryman, all point towards mental discipline and starting early to achieve success. Dr. Bayli points out that if you want to teach Johnny Karate, you better understand karate, and more importantly you better know Johnny, the trainee. Know Johnny's potential and know Johnny's developmental windows so you can him be everything he can be. The *Karate & Sport for Life* Program integrates the latest in exercise physiology, sports training philosophies and traditional martial arts in the Dojo. Martial arts instructors across the United States know that the "DO" (or "the Way") of martial arts provides the mental discipline which can be a mental framework the student will use to for a lifetime of learning. At each age, or stage, there are certain parts of the body that are in development, and specific exercises and drills can assist or optimize this development.

It is possible to make a strong argument that a karate curriculum with the tenants of *Karate & Sport for Life* will enhance any child's athletic potential for whatever sport they pursue later in life. Karate schools and sports organizations often have their best coaches and instructors only work with the "elite student". Long Term Athletic Development points out the best return on our coaching capital is when we use it with the youngest students. The *Karate & Sport for Life* Program identifies the specific ages in human development when we can contribute the most to a child's future abilities. This is also a model used very successfully for decades in track and field in the Soviet Union's Sports Science Program.

The goal of this chapter is to layout some specific times in a child's life when instructors can make the most difference. Secondly, this chapter identifies a simple approach to work-out plans, shows what the window of development opportunity at each specific age, plans the amount of time a trainee needs for the learning phase, always returning to practicing existing skills and finishing with fitness development.

Windows of Development highlight the core principles of LTAD and the *Karate & Sport for Life* program. If there is a specific period of time in a young person's life when they can gain more depth in a particular area of movement and ability, say balance, then should we not provide a wide range of balance exercises to children in this age group? If immediately after puberty there is a greater potential for developing strength, then why not focus on increased volume of strength training into your core curriculum? These critical time periods and areas of potential are identified in Critical Periods in the Development of Performance Capacity During Childhood and Adolescence.[1]

The breakdown of Learning, Practice and Fitness Development is a suggestion of how to think about organizing the training session. Practice is really the repetition of known skills. Learning is the part of class where we introduce new concepts or teach new movement patterns. The last component is Fitness Development.

ACTIVE START (UP TO 6 YEARS OLD)

Begin with kids from 3-6 years old. These children will benefit from play-like skills and drills within the structure of a traditional dojo.

An early active start in a great dojo will enhance the development of brain function, coordination, balance and social skills. It will also help the improvement of gross motor skills during this highly sensitive period.

One of the most important areas to develop in a child is the foundation for self-discipline. An advantage every karate school has is our history of tradition and etiquette, which provides the framework for discipline. We can use our protocols to establish clear rules and consistency for the child's first experiences in the dojo. Young children desire and need clearly defined rules of behavior and expectation. When we provide this environment, their young minds feel safe and free to learn. Create a safe haven for your student's mind and they will learn more quickly.

At this age we introduce basic bows and etiquette of traditional Karate, so the kids have a good first experience in socialization. Ethics of Sport are found in self-discipline which is developed at this age through the example of the instructor's discipline.

Program design and class plans at this stage focus on learning fundamental movement. Early karate skills are built around the ABC's (agility, balance, coordination, and speed). Add this to your style curriculum.

____

1. *Critical Periods in the Development of Performance Capacity During Childhood and Adolescence, Physical Education & Sport Pedagogy* Atko Viru; Jaan Loko; Maarike Harro; Anne Volver; Livian Laaneots; Mehis Viru

Developmental Windows

There are three periods of motor development that are particularly sensitive to developmental support. This is the first of three important ages in which motor skills development will be enhanced with specific drills.

While we would always recommend motor skill exercise at any age, we should focus more during this period the brain and body are remodeling more than other times, so provide exercise for adaptive changes.

Early endurance development is also important at this age. This is the first of three windows when we can exploit the body's growth stage for gains in cardiovascular capacity and endurance. [2]

Learning

Mental strength and focus come from the early establishment of rules and discipline. Teach the rules and tradition of the dojo. Tell the kids what you are going to do and then do it. Establish the etiquette for your dojo. Start and end every class the same way. You will free their minds to learn buy defining the "class."

Practice

Encourage basic movement skills. These skills do not just happen as a child grows older. They develop depending on each child's heredity, activity experiences, and environment. For children with a disability, access to age and ability appropriate adapted equipment is an important contributor to success. Bodyweight exercises like lunges, squats and push-up/plank holds are appropriate in this sage group, but careful attention should be given to monitoring safe and correct biomechanics, while making the session fun.

Fitness Development

Activity, nutrition, and sleep are important at this stage. Complete development includes sleep and nutrition. "Kids who get less than eight hours of sleep have a 300% higher rate of obesity than those who get a full ten hours sleep."[3] To assist in the learning process kids need to sleep. "Because children's brains are a work in progress until the age of 21, and because much of that work is done while a child is asleep, this lost hour appears to have an exponential impact on children that is simply doesn't have on adults".[4]

----

2. *Critical Periods in the Development of Performance Capacity During Childhood and Adolescence, Physical Education & Sport Pedagogy* Atko Viru; Jaan Loko; Maarike Harro; Anne Volver; Livian Laaneots; Mehis Viru
3. *Nurture Shock,* Po Bronson & Ashley Merryman, Twelve Press.
4. *Nurture Shock,* Po Bronson & Ashley Merryman, Twelve Press.

FUNdamentals (MALES 6-9 YRS. | FEMALES 6-8 YRS.)

Build FUNdamental motor skills in an atmosphere of FUN. The basic skills of karate provide what we call the requisite agility, balance, and coordination necessary for physical development at this age. At this stage we should emphasize motor development over precise replication of karate technique. Include flexibility exercises in every class. Encourage participation in a wide range of sports. For most, strength training should only use the student's body weight, but those with great mechanics and sound supervision can show benefits in strength gains using light weights according to the National Strength and Conditioning Association. The though that it will stunt growth is a long-disproven myth.

Use the discipline and etiquette of a traditional dojo to build a structured environment for learning. The rules of dojo conduct will build an understanding of the ethics in sport.

Each instructor should challenge themselves to build a kid's program around the child's needs and enjoyment, and not treat them like adults. Once the child develops an affinity to come to class, more challenging exercises and skills can be introduced. Then the instructor can point the student in the direction of the more complex adult curriculum requirements.

Erikson's stages of development at this age state that the children are developing their ego around learning competence. They want to be industrious and not feel inferior. Teach them how to be competent. Use karate skills as a learning tool.

Socially, children like to play with others side by side, rather than together – "Me first..." rather than "Let's both do this..." It's a difficult time to teach tactics.[5] Develop simple drills in which the child can succeed. Children need to assert themselves and start taking control of their environment.

Developmental Windows

The second period of motor skill development is ages 8 – 10 years. This is an excellent time to focus on the ABCs of movement and add more complex drills and techniques of karate. In the book *Karate & Sport for LIfe* we have age specific drills in karate to develop motor skills.

During this period there is also a window of opportunity to begin speed and explosive strength training. But all drills and strength development must only be done with the student's body weight if their mechanics are correct.

This is an early optimal window of trainability to enhance suppleness for both genders occurring between the ages of 6 and 10. And yes, kids need to stretch.

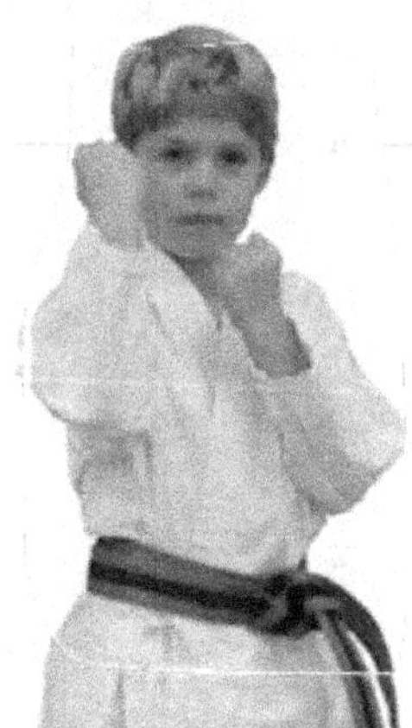

---

5. *The Path to Excellence: A Comprehensive View* of Development of US Olympians who competed from 1984-1998.

Learning

In this stage we work on mastering the general movement skills that will improve the ease with which children successfully learn the more complex, sport-specific skills taught in the later stages of the model.

As you design your curriculum remember these points, Coach John Wooden said, "Never do for a child what he or she can or do for themselves", Maria Montessori said "Never help a child with a task at which she or he feels they can succeed." This age is all about "I can do it".

Competence is extremely important, so design success in your program. Now is the time to start building mental strength.

Basic etiquette and instructor control are reinforced during this phase. The kids love rules if they understand them and the rules remain constant. Remember to free the brain to learn by providing a consistent and clearly delineated environment.

Practice

Teach the ABCs of athleticism: Agility, Balance, Coordination and Speed. Introduce basic flexibility exercises. The development of speed can be done through game-like exercises.

No formal periodization is recommended at this stage, and activities should revolve around the school year with multi-sport camps occurring during school holidays. Regular participation in formal competition is optional but not advised for most students. At this age the most you should do is hold inner-school events or 'friendship tournaments' where participation is rewarded, and competition is not the focus. Children should be encouraged to participate in a wide range of sports at this age.

Fitness Development

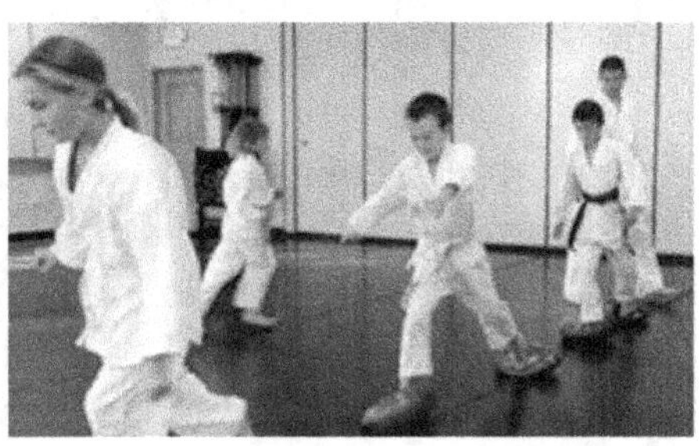

This is about overall fitness to compete to live and be active. Body mind and spirit can be included in fitness. Nutrition is particularly important in these developmental ages along with activity, karate ABC's, and sleep. If you design play-type drills, and timed functional drills, the kids will push themselves to create a more rigorous work out. For children who decide not to pursue life in karate, the skills they acquire during the FUNdamentals stage will benefit them when they engage in any recreational activities and provide a foundation for success in other sports.

Youth sport programs that emphasize fun, enjoyment and love of sport provide a springboard for athletes to continue their development upward.[6]

---

6. *The Path to Excellence*: A Comprehensive View of Development of US Olympians who competed from 1984-1998.

LEARN TO TRAIN (MALES 9-12 YRS. | FEMALES 8-11 YRS.)

Focus on the integration of fundamental movement skills and karate technique. This age group will go through a period of accelerated adaptation of motor coordination. At this age, children are developmentally ready to acquire the general techniques of karate, which will also provide a foundation for fundamental movement in any sport.

This is the stage prior to PHV, (Peak Height Velocity)[7], is commonly referred to as the "growth spurt" in a young person's life. In anticipation of this growth spurt, activity, sleep, and nutrition are very valuable.

This is a critical period for motor development and endurance. At this age, the child is ready to learn correct technique. Discipline and etiquette in the dojo continue which will assist in developing mental toughness.

From ages 8-11 in girls and 9-12 in boys to the onset of the growth spurt, children are ready to begin proper strength training and increased volume in proper karate technique. Prior to this, if kids got the general pattern in kata that was fine. But now we can begin to refine the movement for correct display of karate skills.

While it is often tempting to over-develop "talent" at this age through excessive karate sport training and competition, this single-sport approach can be very detrimental to later stages of development if the child is playing a late specialization sport, like Karate. It promotes one-sided physical, technical, and tactical development and increases the likelihood of injury and burnout, while promoting lesser degrees of athleticism.

Kids at this age should be encouraged towards competition judiciously. Some kids have the mental make up to go out and compete and understand that is about personal improvement and not exclusively winning. Parents love their children and want them to win everything, so it is important to ensure that everyone is aware that winning at this age is good, but development of skill and athleticism is a higher priority.

Apply a ratio of 70% training to 30% competition. The 30% dedicated to competition includes tournaments and your tournament technique training. Long term studies reveal that athletes participating in this preparation for competition are better prepared in both the long and short term than those who focus on winning at this age. This does not mean you should not have the kids compete, just that competition is about the process and the work. The Sensei makes the value declarations he/she appreciates the efforts of the student.

Windows of Development

One of the most important periods of motor development for children is between the ages of 9 and 12. This is a window of accelerated adaptation to motor coordination. This is also a period of accelerated brain maturation, which may also influence improvements in peak muscle power because of improved neural control of muscle activity.

---

7. *Sport System Building and Long-term Athlete Development in British Columbia,* Istvan Balyi Ph. D

Aerobic capacity accelerates from 11 to 14 years. So, encourage adaptive changes by developing more rigorous training and conditioning opportunities. Proper strength training is highly recommended.

Learning

As an instructor you will want to give your students every chance to succeed. You can do this by recognizing that teaching mastery of basic karate movements for your style and emphasizing skill development over teaching competition success, will give them greater long-term satisfaction. Karate is a late specialization sport. Early specialization in late specialization sports like Karate can be detrimental to later stages of skill development and to refinement of fundamental sport skills. At this stage, children are developmentally ready to acquire the basic karate skills and combine these techniques with fundamental movement skills.

Practice

At this age some students that are developmentally older will be ready for a class focusing on practice and less on games. The students that are developmentally younger will need to be taught in the previous stage's environment. You cannot treat all the students the same or lump them in classes based on chronological age alone.

Fitness Development

Strength-to-mass ratio becomes a limiting performance factor during the growth spurt years. Kids that gain weight and change the length of their levers can become "awkward" trying to move the increased mass with a different mechanical system. Bodyweight strengthening exercises should be a part of every athlete's program, and many can now benefit from increasing resistance loads with dumbbells, medicine balls, kettlebells, or bars. Sleep and proper nutrition are also critical for rejuvenation after the increasingly higher volume of work during this stage. Remember, that karate participants during this stage are learning to train, both on-mat and off-mat.

Develop a karate training work-out program that emphasizes a strong anaerobic base, with an aerobic component, through work with interval training. This is probably the most critical stage of development. Physical development, mental/cognitive development and emotional development all go through dramatic changes during this stage.

On mat, move to the next level of the complexity for the ABCs. Integrate the Five S's: (Stamina, Strength, Speed, Skill, Suppleness) into your class plan. Blend karate practice with rigorous exercise. In some karate programs the instructor will simply increase the volume of exercise. But that is only one of five parameters of exercise to consider, (the other four are intensity, frequency, density, and rest)[8]. A great karate program integrates all of these components with a traditional karate curriculum.

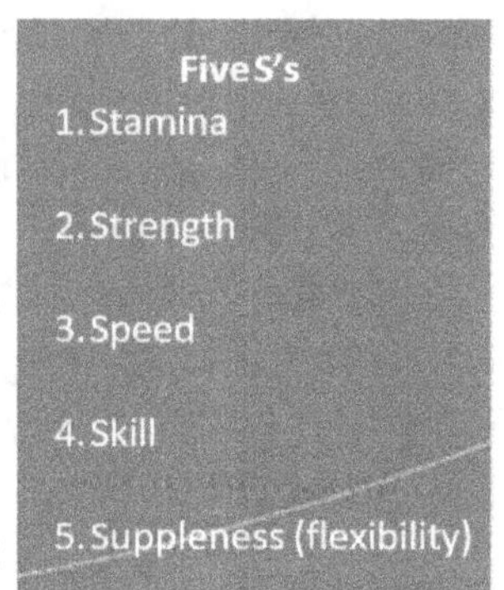

The growth spurt during this period that occurs in most young people is a defining point on how we plan our karate and exercise program. Typically, prior to this growth spurt they are kids, and after the growth spurt, (also identified as the PHV), their young bodies are ready for a consolidation of karate skills and exercise into a program focused as a more adult curriculum. During this age, the student reaches the peak development of speed, aerobic velocity, and strength, meaning there is more significant gains in these areas during this period than any other time.

The *Karate & Sport for Life* Program recommends implementing the philosophy of "Right Practice" as the student becomes mature enough to understand the need for practicing only correct technique. The instructor should press for correct technique, but the coaching philosophy of John Wooden, says to "praise the work, embrace the process, and the outcome will take care of itself." There are a number of books about success and expertise on the best sellers list, all mention this philosophy in one way or another. But it was the founder of Shotokan karate, Gichin Funakoshi, who said "It is not victory or defeat that is important, but the perfection of the characters in the contest we seek."

During these stages, we make or break the karate student, the athlete.

Windows of Development

Explosive strength develops rapidly if stimulated during this period. Calculations based upon creatine excretion indicate that in males from the age of 7 to 13.5 years demonstrate muscle mass increases of 0.6% per year then from ages 13.5 - 15.5 years the increase amounts to 29% per year (Malina, 1969). With explosive strength comes a window of trainability for speed training.

The third window of optimal trainability for aerobic endurance occurs at the onset of PHV. Shortly after PHV aerobic intensity should increase. This can be called aerobic capacity trainability from age 12 to 14 years. (D.S. Holm, 1987)

---

8. *faster better stronger*, Eric Heiden, M.D., Massimo Testa, M.D., and Deanne Musolf, Harper publication.

With the sudden growth spurt, the tendons and ligaments are challenged to change as well, making flexibility and suppleness exercises even more important.

Learning

Regardless of whether you are designing drills to teach your kata or building a competition kumite drill you can employ, "Broken Learning, Mistake Driven Learning, Goal Based Learning, Stress Induced Learning."[9]

Learn to cope with the physical and mental challenges of competition. Teach students motivation comes from learning that mastery is from practice. We must teach them the value of practice. Practice habitually, but never as a habit. This practice will improve competence, will drive satisfaction which will push the student toward the "Flow" found in training.

Practice

Optimize the balance of training and competition; follow a 60:40 training time to competition time ratio. Too much competition wastes valuable training time and conversely, not enough inhibits the practice of technical/tactical and decision-making skills. Train athletes in daily competitive situations in the form of practice matches or competitive games and drills. Traditional curriculum should be taught with the expectation of correct technique.

Fitness Development

Make training for explosive power a priority after the onset of PHV while maintaining or further developing levels of skill, speed, strength, and flexibility. Emphasize restoration daily and flexibility training as well.

Consider the two windows of accelerated adaptation to strength training for females. The first occurs immediately after PHV and the second begins with the onset of menarche. For males, there is one window, and it begins 12 to 18 months after PHV. Note: these ages are based on developmental age.

Periodization can be used in planning on mat, and should be used off-mat, but with consideration for school year, and a tournament season primarily from January to the Nationals in July.[10]

---

9. *The Talent Code*, Daniel Coyle, Bantam publishers.
10. The modern meaning of the term "periodization" is largely associated with Tudor Bompa, who has written and invented significantly on this topic in the last forty years. Major contributions have also been made on this topic by Vern Gambetta, Istvan Balyi, Peter Tschiene and Charles Poliquin.

TRAIN TO COMPETE (MALES 16-18 YRS. | FEMALES 15-17 YRS.)

Prioritize your student's fitness preparation. Supreme physical condition, accompanied by supreme mental conditioning is foremost. Performance diminishes immediately when condition is insufficient. Provide year-round training, understand how to use volume and intensity in exercise. There is a Japanese term for intense training, "Shugyo". This can be defined as "austere" or "extreme" training, it is even a form of spirit training.

By now the students have selected karate as their one sport. The training focus changes to 60% competition oriented, 40% to tactical and technique. It is a good strategy to encourage participation in a variety of tournaments, from local friendly tournaments to State and National competition.

It is important to note, "simply exercising harder at this stage is not guaranteed to make the student better, which is why assessments are important. The training must have the correct intensity, volume, frequency, density, and rest."[11]

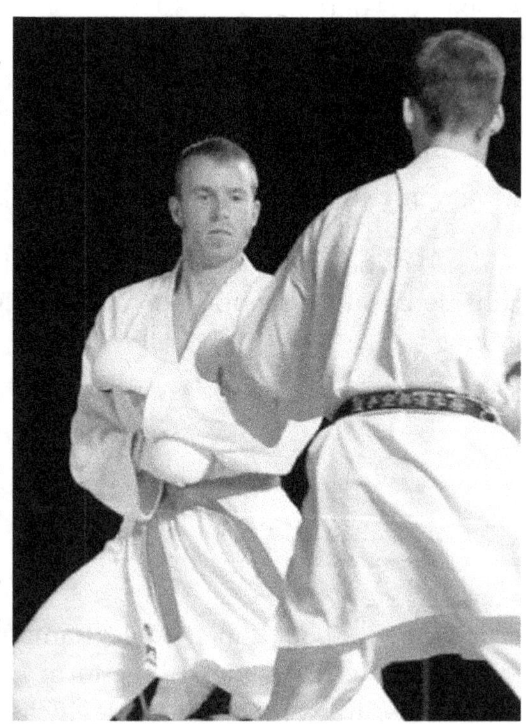

The students in this age group can vary widely in developmental age. A mature young person in this stage can devote 70 to 80% of their time to competition and competition training. A 'late bloomer' will get discouraged if you put them into competition with a much more mature student of the same age.

Hold the late bloomer back, encourage the mature student to compete.

One last note on teaching and training. Improvement in skill from this point on will be smaller and less noticeable so the concept of Kaizen constant and continuous improvement. Small and incremental improvement.

Windows of Development

After PHV, strength training is very important. This is the fourth critical window for motor development. Postnatal, four periods of accelerated brain maturation have been identified. The first occurs between 15 and 24 months of age. The third and fourth periods take place between 10 and 12 years and around 18 years of age respectively (Rabinowicz, 1986; Thatcher et al., 1987). Bio motor ability and trainability (Holm 1987) for maximum strength ages 17 to 18 this is a great window for Aerobic power trainability from ages 17 to 18 years.

---

11. *faster better stronger*, Eric Heiden, M.D., Massimo Testa, M.D., and Deanne Musolf, Harper publication.

Learning

Since the student knows many of the necessary karate skills, learning must become innovative. Use "accelerated learning, risk learning and contest learning". Encourage trainees to explore creation of new drills, combinations and movements.

Continually stress the importance of mental toughness. As Yogi Berra once said, "Baseball is ninety percent mental. The other half is physical." Our mental training program has a great deal of content based on Lt. Col. Dave Grossman's *Bullet Proof Mind*. After all, competition is just abstract combat.

Praise hard work rather than results. In grade school aptitude testing, those who were praised for their effort significantly improved on their next test.[12] The brain is still developing so nutrition support, sleep and exercise are important for myelination.[13] Formal thinking and abstract reasoning develop after hormonal changes. Explanation of our teaching modules are too complex to cover here, but you can find out more in the book *Karate & Sport for Life.*

Practice

Repetition, repetition, and repetition are important under the structure of "Right Practice." Practice must be structured so that skill learning is done while the students is fresh. (See *Karate & Sport for Life*, class organization.)

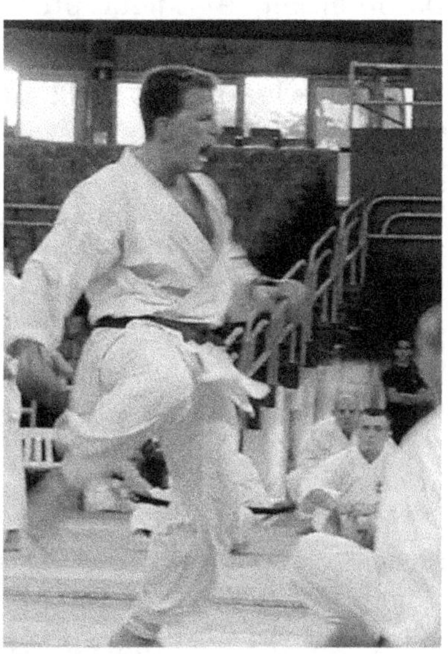

Fitness Development

Strength training drives is the main driver for speed improvement. This athlete should be training as an elite adult in most cases.

Provide year-round, high intensity, individual kata, or kumite-specific training.

Athlete assessments allow you to emphasize individual preparation.

Addresses each athlete's individual strengths and weaknesses. Teach competition-specific training conditioning drills.

In the last stages of puberty, there is an increase in plasma due to growth hormone, making this a strong window for endurance training, ages typically the ages of 14 – 16 years, (Rowland 1979)

Flexibility begins immediately after PHV, and should include PNF, dynamic, and resistance stretching.[14]

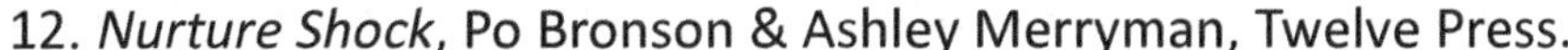

12. *Nurture Shock*, Po Bronson & Ashley Merryman, Twelve Press.
13. *Nurture Shock*, Po Bronson & Ashley Merryman, Twelve Press.
14. *Sport System Building and Long-term Athlete Development in British Columbia,* Istvan Balyi

Transition occurs here as juniors interested in competing can progress to adult competition. The Canadian model uses two stages, "Train to Perform," ages 18 -24 for men, and 17-22 for women, then "Train to Win" men 24+ and women 22+. These two stages have been combined here into one stage, with the caveat that the instructor/coach must be on the lookout for the late bloomers. Students who are developmentally younger should not be pressed forward into adult competition. Since the divisions are arranged by chronological age, the instructor must direct the student to which tournaments will best suit their abilities.

For the student that is mature, this is a perfect age to enter adult competition. Many young men in the Olympic Games, NBA and MLB, and women in tennis and golf are playing at a world-class level in their late teens and early twenties.

This issue is illustrative of one of the "10 Key Elements of LTAD." Developmental age needs to be considered when identifying talent. All of the stages and sequences are delayed in the late bloomer. Since athletic progression is sequential, it is difficult to catch up. You must allow the student to go through each developmental stage regardless of age. We had to learn to crawl before we learned to walk for proper development.

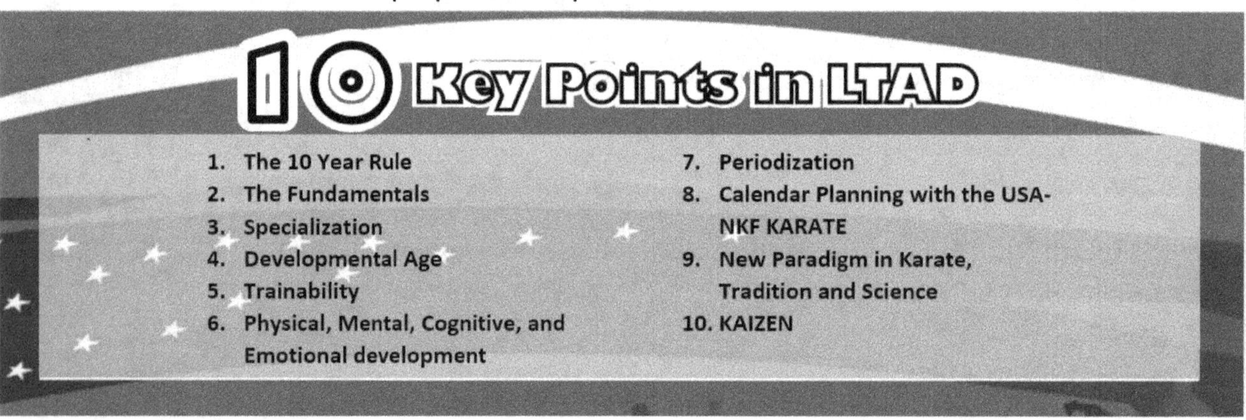

At this age the successful competitors will be interacting with the national team coaches. Our job as instructors is to support all of our students. We can supplement training with modules on N.L.P. (neuro-linguistic programming)[15], motivational psychology, and the social structure of the sport.

Weekly training for elite athletes should total 17 to 23 hours per week and consist of 12 to 16 hours of sport karate training with 5 to 7 hours of karate-specific strength and conditioning. Karate competition training now consumes the bulk of practice. Athletes should also be gaining experience in all areas of international competition in preparation for the "Train to Win" Peak Performance stage. Again, mental imagery is important to supplement training hours.

Double periodization will be applied with tapers and peaks for major competitions and frequent prophylactic breaks. Annual training calendars need to be created on an individual basis. Coaching should focus on ring tactics, performing under pressure. Instructors should learn about

------

15. *Frogs into Princes*, Richard Bandler and John Grinder, Real People Press

IZOF (Individualized Zone of Optimal Functioning). and the OODA. (Observe, Orient, Decide, Act).[16] These are areas of mental response training that have not been fully utilized in the world of sport karate.

Training should be driven by assessments and evaluation of performance in competition. Individualized testing and performance goals can be included every week. Observations and tests should be reviewed with the athlete to build confidence between coach and athlete. Then work together to modify training regime to improve outcome.

Windows of Development

The primary window at this stage is mental maturity/cognitive tactical ability and mental strength with a body that is fully mature it is the mind and mental outlook that will make a difference.

Learning

The instructor creates a climate of mastery and develops drills that drive competence. The emotional social needs of the student will be better satisfied if they are involved in control and choice. The coach should develop an expectation of success and optimism. Direct the student towards understanding "Flow"[17] and developing the SMART Goal Set.[18] Teach accelerated learning though scenarios similar to Futsal, where drill demands simulate or exceed competition demands.[19] Focus on Steady eye movement and postural clues for evidence of mental confidence.

Motivation is not a pat on the back it is real feedback and guidance. After logging 3,000 discrete comments by the legendary coach John Wooden to players, 10% of these were positive, 9% were negative, and the rest the bulk of his comments were information. Short and to the point. A great leader gets great results on simple cues. Those who give lengthy feedback often aren't as proficient or effective.

Fitness Development

Educate the student that they can change their outcome immensely through rigorous training.[20] Maximize fitness preparation and sport, individual and position specific skills as well as performance (maximize engine skills and performance). This is the final phase of athletic preparation. All of the athlete's physical, technical, tactical, mental, personal and lifestyle capacities are now fully established, and the focus of training has shifted to the maximization of performance. Training for competition in this phase is 75%.

---

16. *The Fighter Pilot Who Changed the Art of War*: Robert Coram
17. *Flow*, Mihaly Csikszentmihalyi, Harper Perennial Press.
18. *Mind Gym: An Athlete's Guide to Inner Excellence* Gary Mack, McGraw Hill
19. *The Talent Code*, Daniel Coyle, Bantam Press.
20. *The Cambridge Handbook of Expertise and Expert Performance*, edited by K. Anders Ericsson, Neil Charness, Paul J. Feltovich, Robert R. Hoffman.

Open your dojo to everyone. Our *Karate & Sport for Life* is for everyone. Everyone can make health and performance changes to their bodies. Everyone can be an athlete. Karate has something positive for all.

Anders Ericsson gathered some very interesting information about who is an athlete. We all are.[21] We may not have spent time building the neural circuits, but we can.

In his book *Faster, Better, Stronger*, Dr, Heiden, states, "There is a misperception that fitness belongs to a certain type of person, that exercise is just for jocks. But fitness is, in fact, for everyone. You are exquisitely designed for movement. The human body and brain originally developed, in fact to serve movement."[22]

"Exercise is powerful medicine. It is not just something the US Surgeon General dreamed up to get you out of the house. There are definite, provable biological effects of exercise. We have watched how exercise makes people healthier, often in profound ways. Treat exercise like the powerful drug that it is. Hard, any, or random exercise or simply more exercise is not guaranteed to make you better. To make the greatest use of the shortest amount of time to achieve fitness, you've got to take your exercise prescriptively the right time, in the right amount, at the right intensity, and for the right duration. And no more".[23]

I was recently in Scottsdale, Arizona visiting Ray Hughes' karate school watching a Dan examination. At this exam, there was a very fit, young looking 70-year-old woman, Mary. She led the pace for the young kids. At one point Sensei Ray yelled at Mary for slowing down, prompting Mary to work even harder. There are two important points here, one that you can do this at any age and two that we all need a teacher. Someone who cares about us but pushes us as none of us know what we are truly capable of.

What if you never want to compete or teach your students to compete? In the most sports-focused schools only 20% or less of the students ever compete. So, what about that other 80% of karate students? These people want to feel valued; they want to help. For these people, there is teaching, coaching, and becoming a referee or helper in the dojo or at tournaments.

Windows of Development

It used to be thought that after your 40s, your body would pretty much start to fall apart. Modern science, however, has found that much of this deterioration was more closely linked to people's lifestyle habits, as opposed to deteriorating physiological systems.

You don't stop because you get old, you get old because you stop.

____

21. *The Cambridge Handbook of Expertise and Expert Performance*, edited by K. Anders Ericsson, Neil Charness, Paul J. Feltovich, Robert R. Hoffman.
22. *faster better stronger*, Eric Heiden, M.D., Massimo Testa, M.D., and Deanne Musolf, Harper publication.
23. *faster better stronger*, Eric Heiden, M.D., Massimo Testa, M.D., and Deanne Musolf, Harper publication.

A Harvard Medical School study of more than forty thousand adults that began in 1960 found that exercise along with quitting smoking can add almost four years to your life, even if you start at middle age or beyond. Wolf's law basically states that putting a load on your body makes it stronger; ignoring your body makes it weaker. 14 So the window here is the rest of your life, you can lose 1% of your physical capacities every year, or exercise and slow down or even stop some of the aging process.

Learning

Research during the 1990s, a decade of pioneering brain research, proved that a stimulated mind promotes a healthy brain. The studies were conducted at many research facilities including Harvard, Duke and Johns Hopkins Universities and showed that keeping brains stimulated helps retain mental alertness as people age. The brain's physical anatomy actually responds to enriching mental activities. Scientists have discovered that the brain, even an aging brain, can grow new connections and pathways when challenged and stimulated.

These studies point out the value of incorporating lifelong learning into later lives. Albert Einstein, Claude Monet, Arturo Toscanini, Hume Cronyn, and Pablo Casals, as well as many others, were all productive and vibrant well into old age. Every day that they used their skills and talents to produce great works, they were learning.

Practice

"The striking thing about the work of Anders Ericsson and his extensive study of Expertise is that he couldn't find any "naturals", musicians who floated effortlessly to the top while practicing a fraction of the time their peers did. Nor could he find any "grinds" people who worked harder than everyone else, yet just didn't have what it takes to break into the top ranks. Their research suggests that once a musician has enough ability to get into a top music school, the thing that distinguishes one performer form another is how hard he or she works."[24]

Fitness Development

No matter how old or how young, we can all start a karate program for lifelong fitness. In his book, *Inner Strength Inner Peace*, Tim McClellan tells the story of Bill Robinson. Bill did not start training until the age of 74. He came to Tim, who trains professional and Olympic athletes, and asked if Tim would train him. Tim finishes the story with this personal note, "Without ever saying a word, he has made me vow to keep both my body and mind sharp for life. Through his example I hope to always achieve an acceptable level of resolution in all endeavors, in all areas of my life."[25]

"Setting an example is not the main means of influencing another, it is the only means." -- Albert Einstein

24. *Outliers*, Malcom Gladwell, Little & Brown.
25. *Inner Strength Inner Peace*, Tim McClellan, www.strengthandpeace.com

ADDITIONAL ACKNOWLEDGEMENTS

Growth, Maturation, and Physical Activity. Malina, R.M. and Bouchard, C. Champaign, Ill.: Human Kinetics, 1991

Adaptation in Sports Training. Viru, A. CRC Press, Boca Raton, 1995. 310.p.

Quadrennial and Double Quadrennial Planning of Athletic Training, By Istvan Balyi Ph.D.
Sport System Building and Long-term Athlete Development in British Columbia, Istvan Balyi Ph.D.

Long Term Athlete Development: Trainability in Childhood and Adolescence, Windows of Opportunity, Optimal Trainability. Istvan Balyi, Ph.D., National Coaching Institute British Columbia, Canada and Ann Hamilton, MPE Advanced Training and Performance Ltd. Victoria, B.C., Canada

Developing a Multi-Sport Program, Matt Terwillegar, Utah Sports Summit Presentation, 2009

Early contributions of Russian Stress and Exercise Physiologists Atko Viru Institute of Exercise Biology, University of Tartu, Tartu 51014, Estonia

Learning to Love the Game, Dr. Dan Freigang, presentation materials Utah Sports Summit

Rethinking How we Engage Utah's Youth in Sport, presented by the Utah Athletic Foundation, September 25, 2009

The *Karate & Sport for Life* Program would like to acknowledge the Utah Sports for Life organization, Istvan Balyi & Richard Way, the architects of "Canadian Sport for Life" & Long-Term Athlete Development Strategy (www.canadiansportforlife.ca), from which the underlying sports philosophies and diagrams of this document are based. We also relied on its supplements, 'Developing Physical Literacy' and 'No Accidental Champions'. These internationally recognized best practices will be used as the base of information for the creation of Utah Sport for Life. see http://www.utahsportforlife.com/, for Summer Camps see: http://www.olyparks.com/

ABOUT THE AUTHORS

TIM MCCLELLAN has had a hall of fame career as a strength and conditioning coach, having coached 16 Olympic Champions, over 200 NFL players and World Champions in 9 sports. His passion is training combative athletes. Among those Tim coached were UFC Hall of Famers, World Champion boxers, a World Champion kickboxer, Olympic Gold Medalists in wrestling, the 1996 USA Olympic Wrestling Team, an NCAA National Champion Wrestling Team and National Champions in judo and karate. A martial artist who has earned five black belts, he won 9 individual National Championships in Master's kumite, 4 in breaking and also the Outstanding Wrestler Award at the National Sambo Championships. He has also written 8 books, 45 magazine articles and produced 17 instructional DVDs.

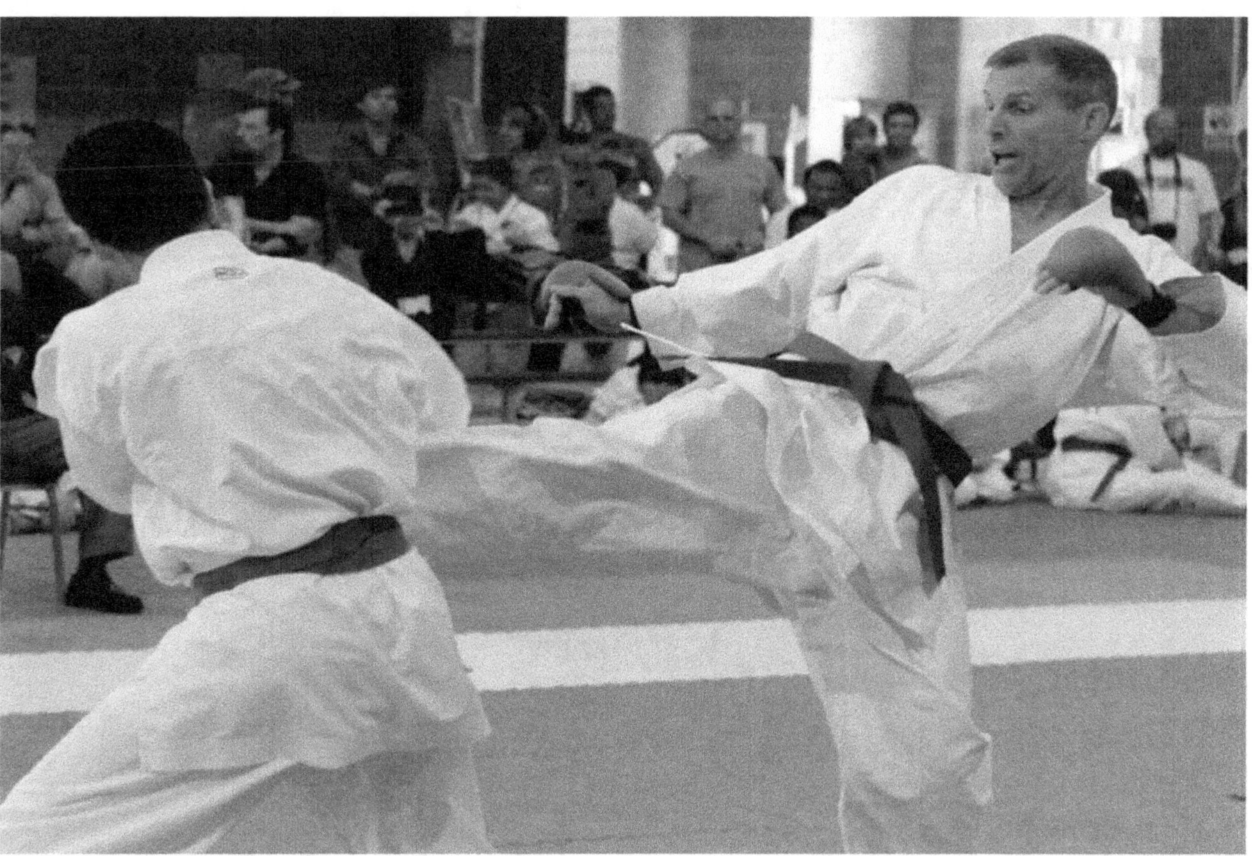

DOUG JEPPERSON has enjoyed a lifetime of high achievement in the combat arts over the last five and a half decades. His journey began in 1966 as a student of American Kenpo legend Ed Parker. This led to an amateur boxing career and NCAA Division-1 wrestling career before he finally settled on studying Wado-Ryu karate under Toshio Osaka. Doug practiced Wado karate for over fifty years, earning Dan ranks along the way from Wado karate founder Hironori Otsuka, Jiro Otsuka, and Tatsuo Suzuki, culminating in a rank of seventh Dan. During his competition career Doug was selected to the USA Wado National Team and medaled in the Pan-Am Championships. As an instructor Doug taught the U.S. Army Special Forces, the Tennessee Drug Enforcement Agency, the Salt Lake City Police Academy and the Utah Olympic Park, among many others. As a sport karate leader, he coached the U.S.A. National team, earned a national referee certification and served on the board of directors and technical committees for both the USA Karate and WIKF-USA organizations. He is the author of *Lifetime Athletic Development* for karate.

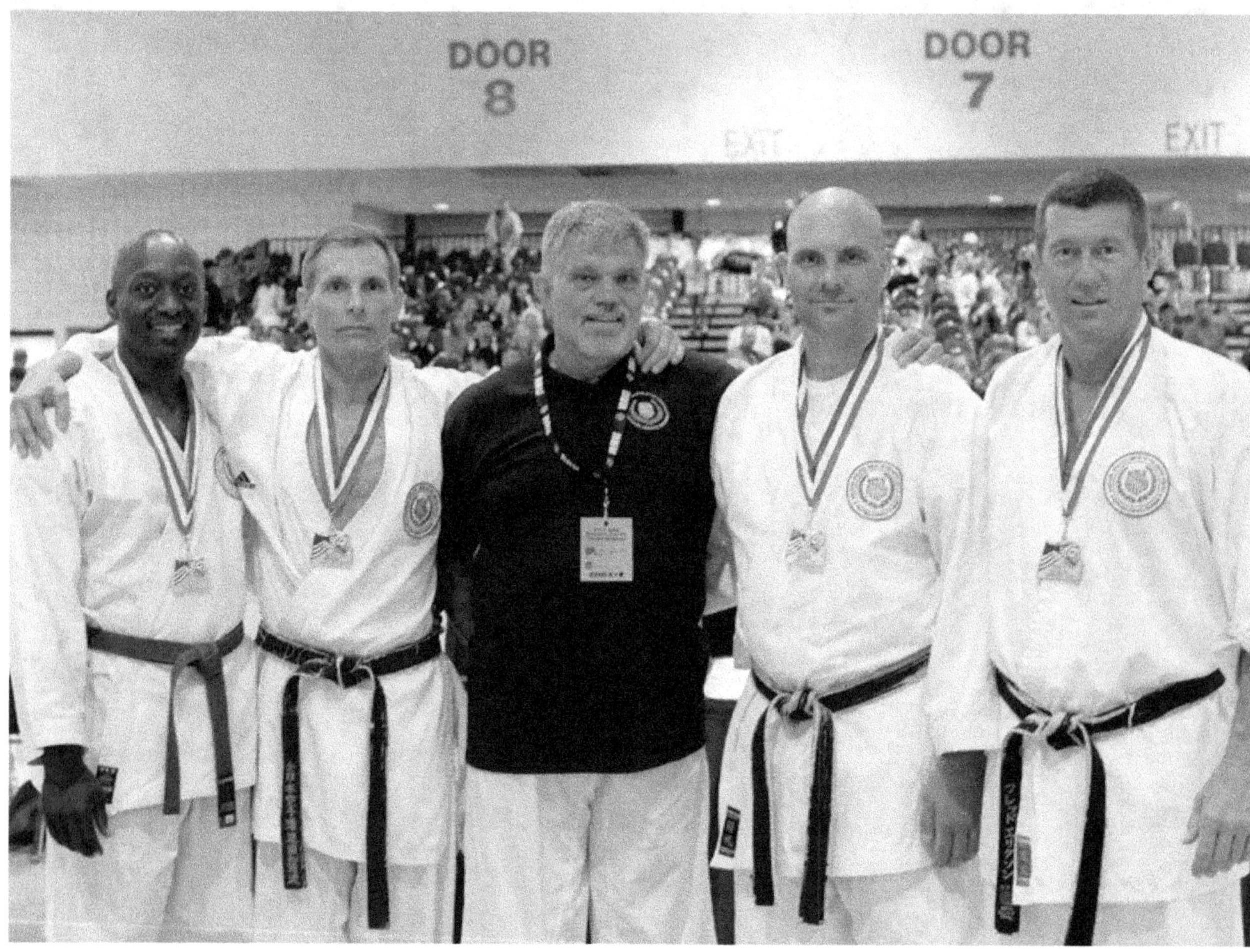